GOD'S Rx

for **FEAR** and **WORRY**

JAMES P. GILLS, MD

SILOAM

Most CHARISMA HOUSE BOOK GROUP products are available at special quantity discounts for bulk purchase for sales promotions, premiums, fundraising, and educational needs. For details, call (407) 333-0600 or visit our website at www.charismahouse.com.

GOD'S RX FOR FEAR AND WORRY by James P. Gills, MD
Published by Siloam
Charisma Media/Charisma House Book Group
600 Rinehart Road
Lake Mary, Florida 32746

Visit the author's website at www.stlukeseye.com.

Library of Congress Cataloging-in-Publication Data

Names: Gills, James P., 1934-
Title: God's Rx for fear and worry / James P. Gills, MD.
Description: Lake Mary : Siloam, 2019. | Includes bibliographical references.
Identifiers: LCCN 2019013546 (print) | LCCN 2019013731 (ebook) | ISBN 9781629996448 (e-book) | ISBN 9781629996431 (trade paper)
Subjects: LCSH: Fear--Religious aspects--Christianity. | Worry--Religious aspects--Christianity.
Classification: LCC BV4908.5 (ebook) | LCC BV4908.5 .G545 2019 (print) | DDC
    248.8/6--dc23
LC record available at https://lccn.loc.gov/2019013546

19 20 21 22 23 — 987654321
Printed in the United States of America

DEDICATION

I dedicate this book to all those who struggle in the war against worry. May each of us find peace by resting and rejoicing in the promises of God.

CONTENTS

INTRODUCTION

I N MY PRACTICE as an ophthalmologist we say that the worst part of cataract surgery is the week before the actual procedure. That's when patients really start to think about the procedure and anticipate its effects. Many patients get concerned at this point about whether the surgery will hurt or whether they will lose their vision. And if they previously had a bad experience with some other procedure, they will be afraid of the cataract surgery.

These concerns and fears are very important and very real. A patient's attitude affects his ability to relax and cooperate with us during surgery so that we can do the best possible job. Therefore, it is essential that we help a patient understand the procedure and that we provide as much comfort and reassurance as possible.

But for some people it doesn't matter how much support we offer. Some patients are going to worry about all aspects of their lives. They're paralyzed by their worries, and they can't enjoy life.

This negative perspective of worry blinds us to the wonderful realities of God's loving care for us. In that state we fail to be grateful for His sovereign rule in our lives. Too often we worry about things that are not a reality and we imagine situations that do not happen. One of the greatest reasons we worry is that we do not appreciate the giver of life or the divine life that He gives us as believers. That lack of appreciation impairs our perspective and disposition more than we realize.

For example, when we are sick, we worry about getting well, failing to realize that God has made our bodies with an estimated thirty seven trillion cells that are actively working to bring about healing. Our worry actually hinders that innate healing process. Our Creator's intelligent design in our DNA has gone before us to prepare the way for our healing. But too many times we are oblivious to His "ever-present help in trouble" (Ps. 46:1) because of our worry and lack of appreciation.

I often ask my patients if they have thanked God for their pancreas today. Probably not, but it has been working for them 24/7 since their birth. And there is much more that God is doing for them and will do for them. Yet their mindset of anxious worry shows a lack of trust in the Lord. It does not reflect a thankful spirit or an appreciation of the Creator and all of His wisdom.

We understand medically that worry is self-destructive. And worry is unnecessary in the light of our faithful and sovereign Lord's care for His highest creation—mankind. Still, we all grapple with it and need to find help to overcome its deadly influence.

Do you know someone who has been paralyzed by fear and negative thinking? Or have you personally ever been so worried that you couldn't think clearly, couldn't sleep peacefully, or couldn't act wisely? This kind of chronic worry is a highly self-infectious *disease* that can permeate our inner beings. It can infect our thoughts, attitudes, and actions. It can destroy us physically and emotionally. Worst of all, it can destroy us spiritually, because chronic worry and fear drive a wedge between us and our trust in God. When we're ruled by negative emotions such as fear and worry, we live in contradiction to our relationship of trust and faith in God. We don't think we can depend on Him. We feel isolated and alone. Instead of resting in the wonderful provisions of His redemption, we blame God for all the bad circumstances in our lives. As a result, we fail to see the blessings He provides.

THE TREATMENT FOR WORRY

Every day we must resist the temptation to worry and fear. I believe the most effective treatment for this destructive disease is twofold. First, we are to cultivate a spirit of thanksgiving as we walk in His love and rest in His redemption. It is in a spirit of gratitude that we learn to appreciate the Creator, Redeemer, and Giver of life. Then, as we cultivate a relationship in profound gratitude for God's sovereignty and His faithfulness, we dislodge our mindset of worry. By trusting in the power and love of God, we learn to live in His peace no matter what situation in life we are facing.

I've seen this twofold treatment work time and again in the lives of my patients. These patients, in addition to facing their own surgery, may have family members who are dying, they may have financial problems, or they may be struggling in a personal relationship. They're certainly sad at times as they grapple with the problems in their lives, but they're not worried.

They're thankful to God for His loving care, and they continually seek His presence in their lives, which allows them to rest in His goodness. They focus in gratitude on all the ways He provides for them. In this place of trust they know He will help them in their pending surgery. Because of their faith they can look beyond their struggles and see God at work continually in their lives. These thankful patients have the same concerns and problems many of us face, but they *choose* not to worry, not to fear. Instead, they choose to be thankful. They have shown me that a constant attitude of thanksgiving breaks the grip of fear and fills their minds with the peace of God.

A thankful spirit

Patients who overcome fear and worry have learned to live the reality of the words of the apostle Paul:

> Rejoice in the Lord always. I will say it again: Rejoice! Let your gentleness be evident to all. The Lord is near. *Do not be anxious* about anything, but in every situation, by prayer and petition, with thanksgiving, present your requests to God.

And the peace of God, which transcends all understanding,
will guard your hearts and your minds in Christ Jesus.
—PHILIPPIANS 4:4–7, EMPHASIS ADDED

When you're focused on the person of Jesus Christ in thanksgiving, your anxieties and fears can be wiped away as your heart overflows with His spirit of peace and joy within you. Paul tells us that a thankful spirit is the proper mindset for all believers. You can reject worry just as my patients who demonstrate a mindset of gratitude have done, rejoicing with thanksgiving in their relationship with Christ.

What a relief to know that all of us can turn our hearts to God and safely put our lives in His hands! We can be grateful for His blessings and let thanksgiving fill our hearts. We can be filled with peace regardless of our circumstances. When we focus on Him with thankful hearts, we can be faithful to the One who faithfully provides.

Appreciation

We have been taught that there are two categories of sin: sins of *commission*—what we do, and sins of *omission*—what we fail to do. My patients constantly hear me say that my greatest sin of commission is worry; my greatest sin of omission is the failure to appreciate the giver and the gift of life. Appreciation involves a sensitive awareness and an expression of admiration, approval, or gratitude. *Appreciate* means "to value or admire highly."[1]

To truly appreciate the gift of life, we must first become aware of the Creator, the giver of all life. Our eternal Creator designed life with a divine purpose. Learning to appreciate the Creator brings us into understanding of His purpose and allows us to focus on that purpose for our lives. As we learn to reverence and esteem our Creator-Redeemer, we are filled with thanksgiving for His benevolence, wisdom, majesty, and power already at work in our lives. We focus on His goodness and love, especially in dealing with the matters that cause anxiety.

Failure to properly appreciate God aborts the possibility of living in the peace of a thankful spirit toward God. Without cultivating that divine relationship, we feel alone, isolated, and totally responsible for our own happiness and success in life. This sense of isolation traps us in self-centered, selfish mentalities, which are destructive in many aspects.

Such mentalities can result in broken relationships, fear, insecurity, and many other unhealthy "syndromes."

A lack of appreciation for God, our designer and giver of life, will inevitably cause us to take all of life for granted. We fail to appreciate not only our lives but also the precious lives of those around us. Like all other sin, a lack of gratitude brings terrible consequences, the gravest being a lack of relationship with God. Conversely, developing a personal relationship with God eliminates the destructive power of anxiety from our lives.

As we learn to appreciate the Creator and His design of all of life, we will seek to know His wisdom as we face life's difficult situations rather than rely on our own confusion of what to do. We will look to His sovereignty, power, and gracious promises instead of our own frustrated perspective. When we learn to deeply admire and appreciate God, we quickly discover that God is much greater than all our problems. We become convinced that when we are worrying, we simply need to focus on God, who will put our anxieties to shame and silence them. It is not always easy to quiet a mind that is "all worked up," trying to figure it all out. But when a fresh vision of God breaks through, the child of God is renewed in his or her soul, receiving new strength to rest in the Lord and enjoy His peace. (See Isaiah 26:3.)

Are you weighed down with worry? Are you filled with fear? There's refuge in the loving arms of God. As you seek to know Him and His love, He will teach you how to rest in His redemption. He will break the bonds of worry. He will banish fear. We get His real and lasting peace when we turn to Him and say, "Thank You, Father, for always loving me. Thank You for the eternity that You offer to me through the person of Jesus Christ, who died and rose again for me." When we turn to Him for redemption, no longer will we experience fear and worry. Jesus promises a life of peace for those who accept His salvation:

> Do not let your hearts be troubled. You believe in God; believe also in me....Peace I leave with you; my peace I give you. I do not give to you as the world gives. Do not let your hearts be troubled and do not be afraid.
>
> —John 14:1, 27

5

Certainly none of us can avoid the situations and circumstances that can create worry and fear. But we can counteract the worry itself by cultivating a spirit of thanksgiving through humble appreciation for our Creator and Redeemer. When we begin to grasp God's greatness, majesty, sovereignty, loving control, and wise purposes, we learn to cast ourselves on His care. As we do, we will see that God has given us many reminders of His precise and detailed attention for our good in all of His creation. This reassures us that God is already at work, not only in creation around us but also in the fulfilling of His promises to us as His children. He is absolutely faithful to those who turn to Him. Therefore, He says to us, "Believe Me!"

In this book we will explore together ways to build our trust in God, deepen our faith, practice a spirit of thanksgiving, increase our appreciation for God, and take practical steps to win the war against fear and worry. The discussion questions at the end of each chapter are designed to help you examine the fears and worries in your life and look at ways you can strengthen your own relationship with God. You may also use the questions as part of a group study to help you talk about real issues within a Christian setting. Additional Scripture verses are included to provide further insight.

Do not fear, for I am with you.

—ISAIAH 41:10

The Bible tells us repeatedly, "Do not fear" and "Do not be afraid" (NKJV). Many of those passages are followed by the words "I am with you" or similar words. It is because God is with us that we do not need to fear. He will always be with His children. May we learn to trust fully in God with thanksgiving for His grace. He will destroy fear and worry! He will give us peace now and forever! Amen!

CHAPTER 1

THE WORRY
DISEASE

MAGINE THAT I got a new sports car. It is just perfect. I love the color and the model. And it came with all kinds of electronic extras and gizmos. It is the fanciest car in the world. But there is one problem: the brake constantly locks on one wheel. Every time I accelerate, I spin around in circles.

While this isn't a true story, it does illustrate how worry affects us as human beings. Worry puts a brake on one of our wheels. We may be the "sharpest sports car" in the world, but we will only go around in circles if worry consumes us.

I know some people who, when they worry, have trouble eating. Others shut themselves up in their offices or homes. In their isolation, worry strangles them. Let me confess that I've spent more than a few sleepless nights worrying about my job, my wife, and my children over the years. I know how worry takes its toll in many areas of life. Let's look at some of its damaging effects.

Intellect

It is human nature for us to take all of life for granted, not stopping to appreciate the wonder of God's creation. Take the human body, for example. It uses its estimated thirty-seven trillion cells to serve us in a variety of ways every day. We are truly "fearfully and wonderfully made" (Ps. 139:14). There is so much that God is continually doing for us—and will do for us—that we simply fail to *appreciate*. This lack of appreciation for our Creator and all His wisdom that He has bestowed on mankind—His highest creation—creates a mindset of anxious worry rather than trust in the Lord when we face difficult health issues or other situations in life that we don't know how to handle.

When our thought processes are cluttered with worry, it affects the way we think. We struggle to have creative and energetic ideas, which results in our producing sloppy and inaccurate work; we end up focusing more on the pressure that deadlines create than on the quality of our work. If anxiety and worry make it difficult for us to eat or sleep, it becomes even more difficult to focus our minds. Disorganization sets in because we can't process information effectively and decide what's important. Distracted, we jump from one task to another with no sense of completion. Indecisiveness results, which leads to non-productiveness. Some people react by becoming workaholics, driven by worries about job or financial security.

When we live in worry and fear, we fail to consider the faithfulness of our God to all who call upon Him in time of need. And we do not understand that He is benevolently sovereign—ruler over all: "The LORD has established His throne in the heavens, and His sovereignty rules over all" (Ps. 103:19, NASB). In our lack of appreciation for God, we fail to receive His infinite love and peace that He offers us freely.

Emotions

We have discussed how our mental health is directly impacted by uncontrolled fear and anxiety. And when we live in constant worry, our *emotions* seem out of control and we do not respond normally to everyday situations. Our worries can turn to fears that produce an uneasiness in us that causes us to be irritable and susceptible to panic attacks. In response, we can become depressed, negative, critical, judgmental, domineering, and controlling. We might be able to manipulate others to be around us, but they don't do it willingly because we're no fun to be with.

Worry and fear and all the negative emotions that arise from this disease can stifle our ability to reach out to others. As a result, we can become less trusting and have difficulty building genuine friendships. We withdraw, getting involved with fewer and fewer people, and eventually become isolated. Anxiety is the basis of many psychiatric and psychosomatic diseases.

Health

Worry depletes us mentally and emotionally and has tangible effects on our physical health. If left unchecked, it can become a progressive disease that can ruin our lives and even kill us. Hypertension is one example of a life-threatening condition sometimes caused by worry, as is a weakened immune system. A weakened immune system makes us vulnerable to everything from repeated colds to much more serious diseases.

Charles Mayo, cofounder of the Mayo Clinic, pointed out how worry affects our entire body, impacting major body systems such as our circulatory system, our glands, and our nervous system, to name just a few. Mayo said he never knew of anybody who died of overwork, but he did know people who died of worry.[1] We can worry ourselves to death, but we can never worry ourselves into a longer, healthier, happier life—a thankful life focused on God.

Thankfulness

In contrast to a life of worry and fear, when we're filled with a spirit of thanksgiving, we are at peace with God and with life. When we learn to rest in God's love and enjoy His redemption working in our lives, we're productive at work, accomplishing a great deal more because we can focus on the task at hand. We know that we are loved and trust that God's loving care is at work in every life situation we face. In this state of peace we eat properly, rest properly, and heal properly. We learn to deeply appreciate those around us and enjoy harmonious relationships with our family and friends. We're able to love and serve others, forgive them, be thankful for them, encourage them, and appreciate them.

The life of Earl Arnett Seamands (1891–1984), a longtime missionary to South India, beautifully illustrates the power of serving others as he lived his life of trust and rest in God. In 1919 he left a successful career as an engineer and moved his family to India to serve as missionaries there. Living in a third world country during the early part of the twentieth century was a daunting task.

Mr. Seamands earned a meager one hundred dollars a month and endured tremendous culture shock in India. Not only were he and his family without things they had taken for granted, such as a piano and a car, but they were also forced to live without running water or indoor plumbing. Unable to make the difficult adjustment to this primitive lifestyle, Mrs. Seamands complained loudly and incessantly. So negative was the atmosphere she created in her home and for those around her that, surprisingly, some of Mr. Seamands' Christian colleagues even suggested to him that he would do well to divorce her.

But this godly man's patient response to their suggestion was, "I can divorce her as you suggest, but that would not be what the Lord would want me to do. I can separate myself from her and her complaining and continue to live the life I want to live, or I can constantly pray for her and become an intercessor for her rather than being her accuser."

In this attitude of humility Mr. Seamands decided to intercede for his wife and assist her rather than resent her attitudes and destroy their marriage. As he continued to pray for his wife, she began to change positively and become more tolerant of their challenging lifestyle. As Mr. Seamands aligned himself with the will of God and allowed his love for his wife to keep him interceding for her, he overcame her critical attitude and continual bickering. As he served her in love, together they triumphed over all odds to save their marriage and strengthen his ministry.[2]

Mr. Seamands' deep appreciation for God and desire to serve Him with a thankful spirit was the focused priority that helped him to appreciate his wife, even though she was behaving in an unlovely manner. His alignment with God gave him strength to overcome the negative situation in his home, surmount the challenges of life during a difficult season, and emerge a stronger servant of God.

MARTHA OR MARY?

In the Gospel of Luke we find two sisters, Martha and Mary, who have different attitudes when it comes to dealing with worry. They illustrate the difference between those who worry and those who don't. In this story we find Jesus and His disciples stopped at the sisters' house to visit and eat. While Martha scurried around the house getting everything ready for the meal, Mary sat at Jesus' feet and listened to Him talk. Finally, Martha was so irritated about doing all the work by herself that she complained to Jesus.

"Lord, don't you care that my sister has left me to do the work by myself? Tell her to help me!" (Luke 10:40).

Jesus' words probably surprised her. "Martha, Martha...you are worried and upset about many things, but few things are needed—or indeed only one. Mary has chosen what is better, and it will not be taken away from her" (vv. 41–42). The problem wasn't that Martha was working. The problem was her attitude. Martha wasn't thankful that the Lord had come to visit with her. She did not appreciate His presence in the way her sister, Mary, did. Martha was worried about the burden His visit created—fixing a meal, preparing the house, tending to the guests. Jesus tried to show her that she needed to change her focus. Rather than giving priority to her work, she needed to give priority to the presence of God.

In contrast, Jesus praised Mary for her attitude. She knew the most important thing wasn't what she did. It was that she was thankful for the presence of the Lord and was aligned with Him. She esteemed Him for who He was and desired to sit at His feet in humility to listen to the words of the Master.

It's the same with each of us. Jesus sees through our work and worry. He knows that what we really need is to change our focus—from anxious activity to reverent relationship. We need to humble ourselves in His presence instead of pridefully trying to "make it" on our own. When we give priority only to our tangible actions and results, such as our work-related activities, without pursuing relationship with our Lord, we'll be filled with anxieties and fears.

When we're aligned with Jesus, our worries vanish. Filled with thanksgiving for His presence in our lives, we are able to see how He guides and blesses us. When we are totally committed to Him, we're engulfed with the presence of God through the person of Jesus Christ, who has promised to give us peace and rest:

> Come to me, all you who are weary and burdened, and I will give you rest. Take my yoke upon you and learn from me, for I

am gentle and humble in heart, and you will find rest for your
souls. For my yoke is easy and my burden is light.

—MATTHEW 11:28–30

Which lifestyle would you choose? Would you rather pursue the
God of peace or be paralyzed by worry? While the right choice may be
obvious, it isn't always easy. Worry starts innocently enough, I think,
as a natural concern about our basic needs. Do we have enough money
to buy adequate food, clothes, and shelter? Is our health good? Are our
friends and family healthy and happy? It is perfectly natural to have
these concerns. In fact it's good that we are concerned because then
we're moved to proper action. We work so we can afford food, clothes,
and shelter. We go to the doctor when we don't feel well. We try to be
loving and thoughtful to our family and friends. And we appreciate
God, expressing gratitude for all He provides.

Satan knows that if we are given the choice, we'd rather have peace
than turmoil, so he uses our own weak human will and desires to lure us
away from our trust in God and into a lifestyle of worry. As we become
less God-centered and more self-centered, our natural concerns become
worries. We quit trusting that God will provide adequate food and
clothing. We believe that we have to focus on meeting our own needs
for the right clothes, the right house, the right car, the right job, the right
spouse, and the right country club. We think we have to take care of ourselves, and we worry about circumstances and events beyond our control. This can lead to selfish behaviors. A mind in this condition is easily
overcome with unreasonable worry and fear and can't tell the difference
between legitimate concerns and problems that exist only in our heads.

None of us is immune to selfishness and the worry and fear that it
creates. It has happened to all of us at some point in our lives. Worry
can have us firmly in its grip without our knowing. The prophet Isaiah
summed it up when he said,

We all, like sheep, have gone astray, each of us has turned to
our own way; and the LORD has laid on him the iniquity of
us all.

—ISAIAH 53:6

This verse has become a great motivation for me when I visualize it in two ways. First, I see myself going my own way, acting on my own dreams, aspirations, and desires. Then I see Christ on the cross, bearing my sins. In the first scene I'm enjoying my sinful pleasure and not caring about God. In the other scene Christ is caring about me and bearing the penalty for my sins.

The first scene breaks my heart even as it challenges me. The second scene provides strength of motivation that comes from the realization that God loves me to such an amazing degree. This realization binds my heart to Him so much that I want to be loyal to Him. When I find myself falling into selfish worry, I go to this verse and envision Christ's great love for me, and as I do, I begin again to trust in God with renewed strength and put aside my selfish ways in order to seek His will.

Will you do that with me now? Pray with me:

> *Lord, I am selfish. I have sought my own way and ignored You. Forgive me when I try to live by worldly standards. Forgive me for thinking that I can't depend on You. I commit myself again to seeking Your will and not the ways of the world. I know that I am Your child and that You will take care of me. Thank You for Your endless fountains of love, mercy, and grace. Thank You for the strength that comes from trusting in You. Amen.*

The following chart illustrates from Scripture the difference between the mindset of worry and the mindset of peace and thanksgiving.

Worry	Thanksgiving
But the worries of this life, the deceitfulness of wealth and the desires for other things come in and choke the word, making it unfruitful. —MARK 4:19 (Worry keeps us from listening to God.)	I will listen to what God the LORD says; he promises peace to his people. —PSALM 85:8 (We listen to God.)

Worry	Thanksgiving
If you bite and devour each other, watch out or you will be destroyed by each other —GALATIANS 5:15 (Worry causes poor relationships.)	Let the peace of Christ rule in your hearts, since as members of one body you were called to peace. And be thankful. —COLOSSIANS 3:15 (We have peaceful relationships.)
The way of peace they do not know. —ROMANS 3:17 (Worry destroys peace.)	You will keep in perfect peace those whose minds are steadfast, because they trust in you. —ISAIAH 26:3 (We have internal peace.)
Cursed is the one who trusts in man.... That person will be like a bush in the wastelands. —JEREMIAH 17:5–6 (Worry dries us up spiritually.)	The eternal God is your refuge, and underneath are the everlasting arms. —DEUTERONOMY 33:27 (We feel God's provision.)
The seed that fell among thorns stands for those who hear, but as they go on their way they are choked by life's worries...and they do not mature. —LUKE 8:14 (Worry makes us unproductive in our work for the Lord and otherwise.)	Trust in the LORD with all your heart and lean not on your own understanding; in all your ways submit to him, and he will make your paths straight. —PROVERBS 3:5–6 (We are productive under God's guidance.)
"Martha, Martha," the Lord answered, "you are worried and upset about many things." —LUKE 10:41 (We are frazzled in our work.)	Trust in the LORD.... Take delight in the LORD.... Commit your way to the LORD.... Be still before the LORD and wait patiently for him. —PSALM 37:3–5, 7 (We have peace in our work.)

Worry	Thanksgiving
Do not love the world or anything in the world.... The world and its desires pass away, but whoever does the will of God lives forever. —1 JOHN 2:15, 17 (We're focused on the material world.)	Though outwardly we are wasting away, yet inwardly we are being renewed day by day. —2 CORINTHIANS 4:16 (We're focused on eternity.)
Their father Jacob said to them, "You have deprived me of my children. Joseph is no more and Simeon is no more, and now you want to take Benjamin. Everything is against me!" —GENESIS 42:36 (We miss God's purpose.)	And we know that in all things God works for the good of those who love him, who have been called according to his purpose. —ROMANS 8:28 (We know God is in control.)
I have no refuge; no one cares for my life. —PSALM 142:4 (We feel alone and isolated. We don't sense God's presence.)	So do not fear, for I am with you; do not be dismayed, for I am your God. —ISAIAH 41:10 (God is with us.)

Worry isn't a permanent state of life when we allow God's Spirit to work in our lives. Jesus came to give us His peace; that's good news for us sinners! In the next few chapters we'll look more closely at the various forms selfishness takes and the different ways it creates worry. We'll also see God's plan for redeeming us from selfishness and helping us surrender to His will. And we will understand how meditating on the wonders of God's creation all around us can evoke deep appreciation and strengthen our trust in God.

DISCUSSION 🌿 QUESTIONS

1. What are you worried about now? How is it affecting your health?
How is it affecting your relationships?

....

....

....

....

2. What makes you feel peaceful? How does that attitude affect your
health and relationships?

....

....

....

....

3. How can you deepen your appreciation for God and for His gracious gift of life?

....

....

....

....

4. List some ways to practice being thankful this week. For example, say thank you to someone you encounter today—a sales clerk, a receptionist, or a neighbor. Or write a note to someone special.

5. What are some of your obstacles to asking God for His peace?

6. What Scripture speaks to your heart about your worries?

CHAPTER 2

AWE, APPRECIATION,
AND ADORATION

A S I MENTIONED earlier, the spirit and practice of thanksgiving is a powerful weapon against the self-destructive "disease" of worry—a disease that we are all too prone to suffer. Why are we so vulnerable to worry? Many people are not living a life of thanksgiving, as we discussed, because they do not truly appreciate the gift of life they have been given. When we fail to appreciate God, it follows that we do not appreciate His gift of life to us—and to others.

The result of failing to cultivate an intimate relationship with our loving God is that we fall into selfish living, seeking only to please ourselves while making unfair demands on others. In our self-centered blindness, failing to acknowledge God, we think our security, our happiness, and our well-being depend on us alone. When we cannot control circumstances and people in order to secure our perceived happiness, anxiety and worry begin to plague our hearts and minds. Without a revelation of God's great power and love for us personally, we can never learn to truly appreciate the gift of life that God has graciously given us to enjoy. In her book *Radical Gratitude*, Ellen Vaughn comments on this sad reality:

> We live in a land that has largely lost a sense of holy reverence, let alone the transcendent. Most everything is assessed by the

criterion, "How does it affect me?" In a supremely self-referential culture, it's hard to conceive of anything that is so wholly Other.... Far too often we trivialize the holy, perceiving God as an extension of ourselves. God is white, just like us. Or black, or Asian, or Hispanic, or whatever.... No. God is huge. Mysterious. Multidimensional.[1]

It is a habit of grateful people, Vaughn concludes, to "look up and see God as God. When we look up to Him, we are first overwhelmed and awed, then full of gratitude that One so huge would deign to love ones so small."[2]

We must recognize, and then that gratitude to God serves as a catalyst to greater appreciation for the gift of life He has given us. Remember that we defined *appreciate* earlier to mean simply "to value or admire highly." I am convinced that if we pause to appreciate God's creation, which is all around us, our selfish perspective of life can be changed. The Scriptures confirm that we can see God in His creation: "For since the creation of the world God's invisible qualities...have been clearly seen, being understood from what has been made, so that people are without excuse" (Rom. 1:20).

As we allow our hearts to be filled with *awe* for the miraculous cosmos around us and the divine handiwork that we are as human beings, we begin to bow in gratitude for God's great kindness to us. We become aware of His great faithfulness and learn to rest in His sovereign rule over our lives. In this way true appreciation for God and His creation can rid us of our worry and anxiety. We begin to comprehend the great love God has for us and learn to cultivate relationship with Him. Instead of our complaining and negative attitudes, appreciation for God leads our hearts to the spontaneous response of *adoration*, filling us with praise and thanksgiving for His gift of life—now and for eternity.

Knowledge of creation reveals to us the nature of our Creator. As we take time to appreciate the world around us and to allow the wonders of creation to fill us with awe, we behold the Creator's infinite hand in our universe. This in turn brings an understanding that He is outside of time or any other finite, limiting force. He is eternal. And if He designed life with a divine purpose, He must desire to reveal His loving eternal purpose for our lives.

Learning to appreciate the Creator can be a beginning point to unlocking for us the eternal benefits of knowing God; receiving His Son, Jesus Christ, as our Savior; and thereby experiencing the infinite quality of life that is eternal. Jesus prayed to the Father that He would give eternal life to all those God had given Jesus. "Now this is eternal life: that they know you, the only true God, and Jesus Christ, whom you have sent" (John 17:3).

Yet it has been my observation that even people of faith—born-again believers in Christ who love their Creator-Redeemer—often lack a profound appreciation for His creation. This lack of appreciation keeps them from fully enjoying the quality of eternal life they have been given in this life. With complaining hearts they fail to comprehend the wondrous gift of beauty in nature. And often in taking their own lives for granted, they abuse the gift of physical health He has given them.

Surrendering our lives to our awesome Creator–Redeemer allows us to enter into His wonderful, divine purpose for our lives. As we express our gratitude to God, our hearts are humbled and filled with appreciation for who He is. The disease of worry is suffocated and displaced when a believer's heart is filled with adoration and worship of God.

The psalmist demonstrates how our humble adoration for God brings the deepest satisfaction a human heart can know.

> O LORD, how many are Your works! In wisdom You have made them all; the earth is full of Your possessions....I will sing to the LORD as long as I live; I will sing praise to my God while I have my being. Let my meditation be pleasing to Him....I shall be glad in the LORD.
> —PSALM 104:24, 33–34, NASB

You probably have a favorite nature scene or sound that fills your heart with awe, if only for a moment. Perhaps it is a special place in nature where you love to breathe deeply and meld your psyche with the view of God's creation in which you are reveling. Or maybe it is when you look with awe into a darkened sky filled with billions of tiny sparkling lights? Do you enjoy the awesome power of a thunderstorm with its lightning flashes and loud crashes? Perhaps you are fascinated by a brilliantly colored wildflower blooming under a rocky crag where no one else will even see it. The phenomena of nature's wonders seem infinite in number and are exquisite in beauty, filling the observant heart with appreciation.

If there is nothing in your life that causes you to feel thankful, I suggest that you meditate on the greatness of God in creation and consider the words of the psalmist: "The earth is full of Your possessions" (Ps. 104:24, NASB). Doing so can fill you with awe and wonder as you behold with new eyes the handiwork of your Creator. Let your eyes see His creation; let your ears hear the sounds of it; enjoy its fragrance and its touch. Let your spirit be enlarged and refreshed by the exquisite beauty surrounding you during your ordinary day, and you will learn to express adoration and praise to God for who He is and who He has made you to be in His great purposes.

> Know that the LORD is God. It is he who made us, and we are his; we are his people, the sheep of his pasture. Enter his gates with thanksgiving and his courts with praise; give thanks to him and praise his name.
>
> —PSALM 100:3–4

Adoration for God brings our grateful hearts into deep intimacy with our Creator-Redeemer. God responds to our love expression with the depths of His love—"God is love" (1 John 4:8). Only that divine love relationship can truly satisfy the human heart's cry for peace, rest, security, and fulfillment.

When you are willing to quit looking for security and satisfaction in your natural circumstances or in relationships with people and begin to allow *awe* and *appreciation* for the Creator-Redeemer to fill your heart, you will find your life overflowing with *adoration* for Him. And you will know deep within your heart that you have no reason to worry or fear as you continually discover God's unfathomable, eternal love filling your life.

DISCUSSION 🌿 QUESTIONS

1. Do you have a favorite "nature spot"? Does it evoke awe of the Creator in your mind and heart? Describe it and the feeling it gives you.

....

....

....

2. Have you compared the infinite greatness of the Creator, God, with your finiteness? Can you trust His love to have control of your life? What areas of your life do you need to relinquish to His infinite love?

....

....

....

3. What divine attribute of God do you appreciate most? Does that characteristic of God evoke adoration from your heart? If so, how do you express your deep love to Him?

....

....

....

4. If you have not done so, memorize Psalm 23 this week. If you have, recite it prayerfully each day and consider the beautiful picture of God's peace, security, and love that it reveals for those who have relinquished their lives to the Great Shepherd.

CHAPTER 3

REALITY
VS. WORRY

T IS A fact that many of the things we worry about simply are not based on reality. They are based on what-ifs. And even the things we worry about that appear to be real may not be when considered in light of the higher spiritual reality that God offers us. For example, we may feel alone, unloved, and without worth. But if we look to the reality of the truth of God's Word, we will know that those feelings do not correspond with reality for believers who have put their trust in God.

> God has said, "Never will I leave you; never will I forsake you."
> —HEBREWS 13:5

> God is love.... We love because he first loved us.
> —1 JOHN 4:16, 19

Our great Creator, God, has infinite love for His creation. And He demonstrated redemptive love for mankind in sending His Son, Jesus, to die for our sins in order to bring us back into relationship of righteousness, peace, and joy with Him. He has designed us to live in His divine peace, love, joy, and deep satisfaction in relationship with Him. When we are aligned with God's reality, it is very difficult to embrace worry, which is based in fear rather than love. His Word promises, "Perfect love drives out fear" (1 John 4:18).

The grandeur of creation's scientific realities can serve as a catalyst to evoke awe and appreciation in our hearts for God. From the precise parameters of our planet to the faultless functioning of our human DNA, we can learn to appreciate God's power and love revealed in His creation. We can face down our worries by meditating on the wonder of God's power and His sovereign care for all of creation—especially His love for mankind, whom He made in His own image. We begin to understand that God is at work on our behalf just as thoroughly, precisely, powerfully, and caringly as He is in the universe. And in that knowledge, we can learn to rest in the sovereign power and love of our great Creator-Redeemer.

Dr. Richard Swenson is an award-winning educator and best-selling author. In 2003 the Christian Medical and Dental Associations honored him with the Educator of the Year award. He has traveled to over fifty countries and has presented his scientific research to such prestigious groups as the Mayo Clinic, members of the United Nations, the Pentagon, and members of Congress. Dr. Swenson says: "The more we understand about God's power, the less we worry about our weakness."[1] And because God is love (1 John 4:8), we can trust His power to meet our every need. In short, when we focus on God, we learn that we have no need to worry.

In his book *More Than Meets the Eye* (also presented in a fascinating DVD series), Dr. Swenson describes the human body as a "reflection of the brilliance, the genius, the power, the precision, the sophistication of an almighty Creator."[2] As we consider together some scientific facts Dr. Swenson presents about life as we know it, allow your heart to experience awe and gratitude for God's great gift of life in creating the human body.

> There are 10 to the 28th (10 with 28 zeros) atoms in the human body—more than there are stars in the universe. We turn over a trillion atoms every 1/ billionth of a second. And if we examine the subatomic space where the smaller-than-atom particles such as electrons, protons, and neutrons dwell, we find we are perhaps infinite in a subatomic direction. The

scientific theory of 'super strings' (fundamental constituents of subatomic reality represented as strings of energy as opposed to particles) postulates that the most basic building blocks of life lurking in the microscopic sphere of our body are 100 million billion times smaller than a proton particle.[3]

The heart beats two and a half billion times in a lifetime and pumps blood over sixty thousand miles of blood vessels. We make two million red blood cells every second. Put side by side, they would circle the Earth at the equator four times. In our lungs at any given moment we have 150 million air molecules. What the retina of the eye does every one-third of a second would take a supercomputer one hundred years to do. The ear has a million moving parts and in many ways is even more sensitive than the eye. The human brain, at a mere three pounds, "is the most complex and orderly arrangement of matter in the universe."[4] The brain can store the equivalent of 4.7 billion books.[5] And it can carry out one thousand trillion logical operations per second.[6]

Perhaps the most amazing fact of human life relates to the human genome and the DNA. Some scientists have estimated there are thirty-seven trillion cells in the human body,[7] and each cell has DNA in its chromosomes. The DNA in one cell is six feet long. If we stretched out all the DNA from one human body, it would reach one hundred billion miles. Yet the initial single-cell DNA of every human being alive today—over seven billion—weighed together would total approximately one-thousandth of an ounce.

Science has been able to reveal the power, precision, and sovereignty of God, our Creator—and He is impressive. So why do we live in such a stupor, being insecure and anxious? Because we forget (or are not aware of) who God is; in that lack of understanding we fail to trust. It is not that He has failed to demonstrate or teach us but that we have failed to understand. We are dim. We should ask Him to take the dimness of our soul away.[8]

These marvels of scientific reality help us understand our own finiteness and should inspire our hearts to bow before an infinite Creator. Dr. Swenson comments: "Do we have any idea the level of power and precision we are witnessing here? What we need is a new vision of God—the real God—not some vague image...the kind of God who stuns the physicists with symmetry; the mathematicians with precision; the engineers with design; the politicians with power; and the poets with beauty. Don't fear science; God invented it all. And a clear understanding of what He has done only enhances our view of Him."[9]

Dr. Swenson wryly confesses that he asks himself two questions when he arises each morning. First, "Is God worried?" If the answer to that question is yes, he cancels his agenda for the day because it is all over. If God is worried, we are doomed. But if the answer to the first question is no, then he asks himself the second question: "Then why am I worried?" The answer is obvious. We need to enlarge our vision. A greater vision of God's sovereignty and faithfulness will let us see the world from God's view and dispel our anxieties.[10]

Our Creator, God, is continually acting according to His eternal purposes for mankind, for the nations, and for each individual life. As we choose to align ourselves with that divine purpose, we come under His divine protection and experience His great faithfulness to guide us through all of life's changing situations.

Because of mankind's sin Christ came to earth to sacrifice His life for all of mankind, making it possible, through His redemption, for us to become realigned with God. When we accept Christ as our Savior and surrender continually to His will for our lives, we can expect to live in peace with God. And as we focus on the infinite love of God to sacrifice His Son in order to redeem us back to Himself, we will find ourselves being continually released from deeper levels of anxiety and worry. We learn to appreciate God and to trust our lives to Him, resting in His great redemption. The Scriptures teach clearly that as believers, who have the life of Christ dwelling within our hearts, we are not to entertain worry and fear.

> Rejoice in the Lord always. I will say it again: Rejoice!...Do not
> be anxious about anything, but in every situation, by prayer
> and petition, with thanksgiving, present your requests to God.
> And the peace of God, which transcends all understanding,
> will guard your hearts and your minds in Christ Jesus.
> —PHILIPPIANS 4:4, 6–7

We were redeemed by the precious blood of Christ in order that we could live in thanksgiving and enjoy the peace of God, without anxiety. As stated in the Westminster Catechism, "Man's chief end is to glorify God, and to enjoy him for ever."[11] He created mankind in His image and desires that we enjoy intimate relationship with Him and bring glory and honor to His great name. Any doubt we might have of God's great love for us can be put to rest by our understanding of God's awesome creation that He designed for us to inhabit and the amazing complexity of the gift of life He gave to us.

Eternity spent with God will be filled with discovery of the wonder of who He is—getting to know Him and His wonderful works. Yet even now if we seek Him in faith, our daily lives will be impacted with the sovereign power, majesty, and love of God, causing us to relinquish all fear, doubt, and anxious worry. And we will be filled with thanksgiving, bowing our hearts before Him in awe, appreciation, and adoration for His infinite attention to the details of our lives.

These words of Jesus instructed and comforted His disciples to know His promise to them, and they will do the same for you:

> Peace I leave with you; my peace I give you. I do not give to you as the world gives. Do not let your hearts be troubled and do not be afraid.
>
> —JOHN 14:27

DISCUSSION QUESTIONS

1. In what areas of your life does your sense of reality need to be redefined to reflect God's spiritual reality (His Word and promises)?

....

....

....

2. How would accepting God's spiritual reality in those areas of your life change your perspective? Your attitudes? Your actions?

....

....

....

3. Have you considered the scientific wonder that your human body is? How could you bring greater glory to God in your body? Some examples would be exercising, eating well, and giving up destructive habits.

....

....

....

4. What specific steps could you take to align yourself with God's spiritual reality to displace areas of worry in your life?

....

....

....

CHAPTER 4

FAITH
OR FEAR

F OR MANY OF us, our naturally wondrous body, coupled with our attentive stewardship to its well-being and the assistance of caring medical experts, defines all the possibilities for healing. But is all healing related to a physical event in these terms? Or is there something beyond our physical well-being that demands our attention when considering healing and health?

As the crown of God's creation, we are so much more than physical clumps of tissues. We are not only physical but mental, emotional, and spiritual beings. All aspects of our exceptionally designed bodies, minds, emotions, and spirits are integrated into a unified whole, which is greater than the sum of its parts. The completeness of our entire person mirrors this complex life entity. In light of this, how do illness and healing register in regard to the effects they have on our "inner being?"

Scripture tells us that we need to be transformed through the renewing of the mind and aligned with God's design for wholeness through Christ in order to be the recipient of all that He is. Engaging our lives in this integration with God's redemption of our bodies, souls, and spirits requires our total surrender to our Savior. "Not my will, but yours, be done" (Luke 22:42). Our denial of our selfish pursuits presents us to God as a holy, pleasing, and available recipient of all He is. It makes it possible for us to live a life of continual healing—health and wholeness—spiritually as well as physically. We were made to rest in His love and live in harmony with Him in order for our entire being to enjoy alignment with His main purpose, which is to draw us into intimate fellowship with Him.

We are thinking, feeling creations of the Creator, with needs for mental and spiritual healing when godly balance has been overturned in those areas. What is required for this healing of mind and spirit? What are the ways we must seek to align ourselves with God's design in order to be healed? What is God's prescription for our inner healing? It begins with unification of all of our human components—a divine balance and communication among body, mind, emotions, and spirit. This unification, this wholeness and balance at the mental and spiritual levels, is proven to affect the capacity of the physical body to heal.

Mentally we must seek to have "the mind of Christ" (1 Cor. 2:16), which means remaining positive and hopeful and full of faith, and constantly rejoicing with great feelings of thankfulness. Spiritually we must allow God's Holy Spirit to reign in every part of our being. By focusing on eternal life rather than temporal existence, we align ourselves with God and His purposes (2 Cor. 4:16–18), exchanging fear for faith in the Creator. A faith-filled life promotes inner healing of mind and spirit while strengthening the body.

When we speak of physical health and healing, we are referring to maintaining or reacquiring balance of the body's complex systems by adhering to guidelines that the body's design dictates. Physically we align with God's purpose by accepting the stewardship of our bodies, in which He will dwell. When we speak of balance in hearts and minds, we refer to it as *realignment.* That is, to prosper, one must come into conformity with the spiritual principles and precepts by which he or she was created. This is the path toward healing. It is a path toward God. When that is accomplished, we are restored to God's design and His plan and enjoy the peace and joy that He intended for us in creation.

FAITH AND HOPE

Biology plays a large part in the development of personality, as do the social environments we are exposed to from birth. However, we also have choices to make. When faced with challenges to our temporal existence, do we allow fear and worry to take the reins, or do we choose faith and hope over all negative emotions? When we appreciate our fearful and wonderful design, and the One who designed us, through prayer and in faith in Him, hope can rise in even the direst circumstances. One need only ask my friend Dr. James Avery.

Dr. Avery works with hospice patients—those who are dying and have little hope of recovery. He believes that not only is hope a real possibility in one's last days, but it is also a necessity.[1] Now, it is true that the hopes of those facing imminent death differ from the hopes of those of us who are healthy. Those facing death typically hope for a peaceful death, for the well-being of loved ones left behind, and for healing that beats the odds. The important thing is that hope flowers in every heart. It is vital that we comprehend the immensity of this spiritual aspect of healing.

Our Creator endowed us with the inner capacity for hope; it is part of His design for healing and something we must nurture in ourselves and in each other. "The Spirit you received does not make you slaves, so that you live in fear again; rather, the Spirit you received brought about your adoption to sonship. And by him we cry, 'Abba, Father'" (Rom. 8:15).

Fear produces stress, which in turn induces a stress response. This stress response involves changes in the body when one experiences a challenge or threat. The greater the perceived threat, the more intense and comprehensive the response. It is important to note that the effects of the stress response are equivalent whether the threat is real or simply imagined.[2] A broken heart, loneliness, fear, and worry—these all contribute to whatever physical illnesses one may be experiencing and in turn play upon the effectiveness of our healing. This need not be the case though.

Worry, anxiety, and fear exaggerate our physical illnesses and impede our healing. I tell my patients that worry and fear are worse than syphilis. You can treat most cases of syphilis, but it is much more difficult to treat most cases of worry or fear. Our imaginations are powerful, allowing fear and worry to make "mountains out of molehills." A mountain of stress in one's life can make one more susceptible to illness and diseases such as cancer.

Cancer-susceptible personalities tend to suppress toxic emotions such as anger, suffering their burdens in life alone rather than seeking comfort from God and sharing their lives with others. They are also frequently unable to cope with stress. Stress is now known to suppress the immune system, and it does this more effectively in cancer-susceptible individuals, overwhelmingly so.[3]

God's Word tells us that by His Spirit we are able to live overcoming lives. "For God gave us a spirit not of fear but of power and love and self-control" (2 Tim. 1:7, ESV). This means that it is possible for us to displace fear with faith in God. Fear is actually a spiritual disorder that derives from a basic lack of trust in Christ, and as such it is sin.

As we mature in our walk with the Lord, hopefully we come to understand that simple, trusting, abiding faith cannot be easily ruffled. Fear, anger, bitterness, or an underlying sense of insecurity are usually signs that somewhere along the way we have stopped relying on God and have chosen to place faith in our own abilities and independently govern ourselves. When this happens, we find ourselves operating in fear, which leads to anxiety, confusion, and a generally miserable state of being. Oswald Chambers said, "Faith is deliberate confidence in the character of God whose ways you may not understand at the time."[4]

Mark Twain once wrote that courage isn't the absence of fear but the mastery of it.[5] Put another way, courage is the place where fear and faith meet to the defeat of fear and the victory of faith. "Fear has been described as a small trickle of doubt that flows through the mind until it wears such a great channel that all your thoughts drain into it."[6] Even tiny fears that go unchecked can build up into paralyzing trauma. Faith turns off the flow and redirects one's thoughts, allowing a reprieve in the midst of adversity.

MENTAL HEALING

Sometimes we think that the Prince of Peace Himself couldn't possibly relate to the horror and dismay that has invaded our lives. However, in the Garden of Gethsemane Jesus said, "My soul is overwhelmed with sorrow to the point of death" (Matt. 26:38). Scripture says He went and threw Himself on the ground. This is the scene of a straining, agonizing, and struggling Jesus. The Book of Hebrews depicts the scene well: "During the days of Jesus' life on earth, he offered up prayers and petitions with fervent cries and tears to the one who could save him from death" (Heb. 5:7). He truly was "a man of sorrows and acquainted with grief" (Isa. 53:3, ESV). He knows the depths of human suffering as no one else has experienced. And He triumphed over it to bring us the peace of His salvation. Is it any wonder that He invites us into His presence?

> Come to Me, all you who labor and are heavy laden, and I will give you rest. Take My yoke upon you and learn from Me [the precept], for I am gentle and lowly in heart, and you will find rest for your souls [the reward].
> —MATTHEW 11:28–29, NKJV

God does not intend for us to live in fear and endless apprehension. Our fear level is ultimately a referendum on the closeness of our friendship with Him. When God says He'll never leave us or forsake us, He means it! (See Isaiah 41:10.)

Fear is understood to generate from six general categories: poverty, criticism, loss of love, illness, old age, and death. Fear from any one of these can lead to mental disorders that terrorize the mind and cripple the emotions to the point that one becomes bound by guilt, despair, and chronic bouts of anxiety. When this happens, instead of being productive, we lose confidence in our own ability and become ill at ease. If one continues in this frame of mind, it can lead to severe mental disorders such as paranoia. Paul said, "Let this mind be in you which was also in Christ Jesus" (Phil. 2:5, NKJV). That can be a reality, or the scriptures would not instruct us to make it a goal for our lives.

Physical threats are a source of fear that can act on the mind and body to such an extent that the organs in one's body cease to function as God intended. Scripture tells us that King David knew physical fear. As a shepherd boy tending his father's flock, he fought off a bear and a lion. As an adult he lived with the threat of death from King Saul for many years. Yet in the psalms he was able to say, "I will fear no evil," not because there was no evil, but because he had learned early on that God was his protector—"For Thou art with me" (Ps. 23:4, kjv).

There will always be real and genuine reasons for fear. Christians, as well as unbelievers, will suffer physical distress. However, there is freedom from fear of the most ominous threats to our well-being when our confidence is grounded in God and His Word. When we trust in God's wisdom and love, we can live with a fearless abiding in the divine love and redemption of One who has our best interests at heart. A great saint of God who lived in the 1600s, simply called Brother Lawrence, referred to this fearless abiding as "practicing the presence of God,"[7] and he considered it a lifestyle choice.

The Abbe de Beaufort describes Brother Lawrence's epiphany as he heard it in their first conversation together:

The first time I saw *Brother Lawrence*, was upon the 3rd of August, 1666. He told me that God had done him a singular favor, in his conversion at the age of eighteen.

That in the winter, seeing a tree stripped of its leaves, and considering that within a little time the leaves would be renewed and after that the flowers and fruit appear, he received a high view of the Providence and Power of God, which has never since been effaced from his soul. That this view had perfectly set him loose from the world, and kindled in him such a love for God, that he could not tell whether it had increased during the more than forty years he had lived since....

That we should feed and nourish our souls with high notions of God; which would yield us great joy in being devoted to Him.

That we ought to quicken, i.e., *to enliven, our faith*. That it was lamentable we had so little; and that instead of taking *faith* for the rule of their conduct, men amused themselves with trivial devotions, which changed daily. That the way of Faith was the spirit of the Church, and that it was sufficient to bring us to a high degree of perfection.

That we ought to give ourselves up to God, with regard both

to things temporal and spiritual, and seek our satisfaction only in the fulfilling of His will, whether He lead us by suffering or by consolation, for all would be equal to a soul truly resigned.[8]

I have come to know many who, like Brother Lawrence, understand the great benefits of practicing the presence of God as a lifestyle, of giving themselves up to God and seeking satisfaction only in fulfilling His will.

HOPE AS AN ANTIDOTE

Worry and fear can derive from our lack of control in life, or rather a perception of a lack of control. Larry Burkett and Reese Patterson, in their seminal volume *Handbook of Religion and Health*, expressed the need for patients to be informed and to be active in their medical healing process. This involvement includes the thoughts, feelings, and actions (our behavior) that distinguish us from one another. Burkett and Patterson point out that the beautiful thing for the believer is that with faith in God and His hand in every event of life, the sense of control internally, that is within oneself, is enhanced.[9] Such a sense of control, stemming from knowing our loving God is in control, means less stress, greater peace, and therefore a better disposition toward healing.

Negative elements are proven impediments to total health and healing. They undermine and erode the wonderful gift of hope that the Lord embedded in every human heart, often creating hostility and an "enduring pattern of suspiciousness, resentment, frequent anger, and cynical mistrust of others."[10] Unfounded and exaggerated fears often result in such hostility, in despondency, and in a willingness to give up. How can we be healed in such a mental and spiritual state? By living with the hope that comes from God: "But God intended it for good" (Gen. 50:20).

Hope is important, but hope lacks substance until it is rooted in faith. Such hope is birthed and cultivated as we live in an attitude of gratitude, thanksgiving that causes us to live with expectant joy even when we have to wait a little while for the answer. Humans cannot live without hope, without the sense that something good can be attained from the direst situations.

Yet we sometimes lose hope so easily. Why is that? Perhaps it is because we lack the full knowledge of what it means to hope in God. God's Word assures us of His character, and that is why it should become our go-to place in times of trial—so that we can develop a habit of thankfulness toward God and others. Our ability to hope, to search for God's plan within hardship, is central to healing.

Hope is faith talking aloud, drowning out voices of defeat. An example is found in Mark 5:25–28, where we read about the woman with the issue of blood. Hope gave her the tenacity to press forward in faith. The Amplified Bible, Classic Edition, says, "For she kept saying, 'If I only touch His garments, I shall be restored to health.'"

You can energize others with words of hope and encouragement even as you go through your own difficult times. Words of hope sow seeds that bring a harvest. Such words brought a mighty harvest of success to George Frideric Handel, the great composer of the *Messiah* oratorio, late in his career. He drew encouragement and inspiration from the timely words a friend sent to him at a low point in his composing career.

He was a has-been, a fossil, a relic, an old fogy, but it hadn't always been so. As a young man, George Frideric Handel was the talk of England, the best paid composer on earth, and his fame soared around the world.

The glory passed however, audiences dwindled, and one project after another failed. Handel grew depressed. The stress brought on a case of palsy that crippled some of his fingers. "Handel's great days are over," wrote Frederick the Great, "his inspiration is exhausted." Yet his troubles also matured him, and his music became more heartfelt. One morning Handel received a collection of various Biblical texts from Charles Jennens. The opening words from Isaiah 40 moved Handel: "Comfort ye my people."

On August 22, 1741, he began composing music for the words. Twenty-three days later, the world had Messiah, which opened in London to enormous crowds on March 23, 1743. Handel led from his harpsichord, and King George II, who was present that night, surprised everyone by leaping to his feet during the "Hallelujah Chorus." From that day audiences everywhere have stood in reverence during the stirring words: "Hallelujah! And He shall reign forever and ever."[11]

You can't hold back a man or woman whose hope is in the Lord. To that person, God is always bigger than the giants that threaten to keep you out of the promised land. Saturating our souls in His Word enables us to rise above despair. Caleb and Joshua saw the giants in the land but knew that with God they could overcome (Num. 13). The prophet Jeremiah looked at the smoldering ruins of Jerusalem and responded in much the same way. He had the devastating facts, yet in the midst of the lament he reminded himself of the reliability and faithfulness of the God he served.

> This I recall to my mind, therefore I have hope. Through the LORD's mercies we are not consumed, because His compassions fail not. They are new every morning; great is Your faithfulness. "The LORD is my portion," says my soul, "Therefore I hope in Him!"
> —LAMENTATIONS 3:21–24, NKJV

As we receive God's Word through faith, hope rises within us, dispelling disappointment and confusion. When we become living epistles, those who see our witness can receive God's living, life-giving hope just as they receive it by reading His written epistles. Our faith anchored in Him enhances the faith of others. Joyous faith founded in hope cannot be explained, but it is "an anchor of the soul, both sure and steadfast" (Heb. 6:19, NKJV).

DISCUSSION QUESTIONS

1. What do you do when you experience feelings of hopelessness?

_____

_____

_____

_____

_____

2. Does knowing God and being able to trust Him help to restore your hope? Explain how.

_____

_____

_____

_____

_____

3. Read Hebrews 11:1 and 1 Peter 1:7–8. Write in your own words what these New Testament writers were trying to convey about hope.

_____

_____

_____

_____

_____

CHAPTER 5

A NEW
PERSPECTIVE

ACH OF US is tempted by coveting what the world values. For some it's clothes or cars. For others it's a relationship or a career. All of us battle selfish desires to see, measure, and own the tangible possessions of the world. Jesus says in Mark 4:19, "The worries of this life, the deceitfulness of wealth and the desires for other things come in and choke the word, making it unfruitful."

Worry comes from the Old English term *wyrgan*, which carries the connotation of "to choke or strangle."[1] Worry can creep into our lives and strangle us. Do you worry about keeping your possessions, health, status, or position in life? Jesus tells us to change our focus.

> Do not store up for yourselves treasures on earth, where moths and vermin destroy, and where thieves break in and steal. But store up for yourselves treasures in heaven, where moths and vermin do not destroy, and where thieves do not break in and steal. For where your treasure is, there your heart will be also.
> —MATTHEW 6:19–21

We are not to concern ourselves too much with earthly goods. Instead, our Good Shepherd tells us to be more concerned about eternal treasures. How can we do this? We can look at this world through eyes focused on the eternal God, who enables us to see His blessings, appreciate Him for who He is, and live humbly grateful for the gift of life He has given us. When this happens, our hearts are filled with His love and we desire to return that love in worship and adoration to Him. Our focus shifts from material possessions to loving and serving God with thanksgiving every day and letting that love guide our actions and attitudes in our relationships with others. Being aligned with God helps us care for others—a sure antidote to selfishness.

It's natural to be concerned about having adequate food, shelter, and clothes. But when the worldly values of always pursuing "more" creep into our thinking, we've chosen earthly treasures over the heavenly. We've chosen to turn our backs on God's Word, creating a void in our lives. The world tells us the way to fill the void is by getting more from our profession, relationships, appearance, status in life, money, and possessions.

Even those who "have it all" worry about keeping what they have and about getting more. They worry about whether they can trust others, because they think everybody is just looking out for themselves. They worry about making the right impression on the right people so others will think they are important. Instead of having it all, all of it has them.

God wants to give us a new vision of life. Think of it as our Father owning the land on both sides of the river. One side is the present; the other side is eternity. We will be eternally cared for by Him. There is nothing we could want that He can't provide. This kind of freedom from want frees us from worry and fear. We have no fears of loss or even death because He has promised to let us live in His presence forever. We have the freedom of that eternal bliss of being engulfed with Him.

> So we fix our eyes not on what is seen, but on what is unseen,
> since what is seen is temporary, but what is unseen is eternal.
> —2 CORINTHIANS 4:18

ADORATION

While earthly treasures are fleeting, living in the presence of God lasts for eternity. Thanks be to God for the bliss of eternity we have to look forward to with Him! It is this eternal perspective and hope that fill our hearts with adoration for our Creator-Redeemer. Adoration is the spontaneous heart response to a revelation of our eternal God, who desires intimate relationship with His children. Adoration for our God fills us with praise and thanksgiving for His gift of life. It is in this posture of worship that we conquer fear and worry. It is there that we learn what it really means to rest in His redemption, desiring to glorify God and enjoy Him forever. Adoration also brings us to repentance for our great sin of omission—a lack of appreciation that takes all of life for granted.

When we go beyond this life into eternity, the bliss that awaits us is indescribable. Our Father has given us His eternal kingdom. In light of that wonderful spiritual reality the importance of everything else pales in comparison. Of no importance are the jobs we have or the possessions we own. Of great importance are the eternal matters—such as our home with God in heaven. Our earthly possessions are His blessings, and we should praise Him for giving us such gifts. But our true home, our true security, is found in relationship with the person of Jesus Christ. Being a member of His kingdom gives us a place, beginning now and lasting through eternity.

To cultivate this kind of eternal perspective, we need to adjust our temporal priorities, being content in earning enough to meet the needs of our daily lives without allowing those needs to consume our thoughts and energies. As we place our focus on our eternal future with God, we become consumed with a *future* that begins *now*, enjoying His eternal presence in our daily lives. We bow our hearts in worship and adoration for His love, His faithfulness, and His sovereign care in our lives. In that way we live in anticipation of heaven, of spending eternity in His presence. And we make our life decisions based on that perspective. Martin Luther said, "I live as though Jesus died yesterday, He rose today and is coming back again tomorrow."[2]

AN ETERNAL PERSPECTIVE

Think of Jesus as dying only yesterday. Calvary was yesterday. The power of the resurrection is manifest today. The power we live by today is the Holy Spirit. We live with Jesus today. Tomorrow we look forward to living in His grace for eternity.

In Matthew 6:25–33 Jesus is explicit in His instruction not to worry. He puts our concerns in proper perspective. We are of much greater value than the birds and flowers that God takes care of. We have nothing to fear because the Lord knows what we need, and He will give it to us, now and for eternity. This reality should humble us and fill our hearts with deep appreciation for the loving care of our heavenly Father. As we express our thanksgiving and gratitude for His love, our hearts are filled with His peace.

Jesus wants us to be free from the worries and anxieties that can rule our daily lives. He wants us to see our lives from God's point of view, not man's. He wants us to see the world around us as short-lived, our problems as temporary. He wants us to take our focus off our own needs and desires and plans and not think by the standards of this world, focusing instead on eternity in His presence.

God will take care of our problems; all we need to do is rest in His presence. When we understand that, how can we worry about the events and circumstances of this world? We have all of eternity with Christ stretching out before us.

Dietrich Bonhoeffer, a renowned theologian, faced execution by the Germans during World War II. His response to that inevitable fate was simply, "This is the end, but also the beginning."[3] Each of us can live with the anticipation of heaven in our hearts. His presence is relevant to every aspect of our daily lives—our jobs, our relationships, our mental thoughts and attitudes, our rising in the morning and resting at night, and our continual thanksgiving for that eternity.

This eternal perspective has practical applications. Here are five steps each of us can take to diagnose and analyze our worries.

1. **Take one day at a time.** "This is the day the LORD has made; we will rejoice and be glad in it" (Ps. 118:24, NKJV). We are often so busy smothering the present moment with worries about tomorrow or regrets about yesterday that we kill today. Don't worry about tomorrow or six months from now. Don't worry if the

government is going to take over the medical system or if social security is going to go broke. We just need to do the very best we can where we are with what we have. Don't worry about the rest. Tomorrow belongs to God. We have no control over the future, but He has promised to provide for us eternally. We have only today; let us enjoy it and be thankful.

2. **Get the facts.** Write down all the information you have about the situation you're worried about. Keep a list on paper, not in your head. Not everything comes quickly. Write down all the details, and analyze them. "What exactly is it that I'm worried about? What are the consequences? How does it really affect me?" As we write down our worries, we become followers who trust in God to provide and who see Him at work.

3. **Analyze the results.** As we think through a worrisome situation, we often realize it's not the event that troubles us—it's the anticipation of the event. We realize certain things are going to happen regardless of what we do. Those that can't be cured must be endured. And we can endure them because we know God is in control now and for eternity. Our attitude of thanksgiving will help us put Him first and trust in His goodness and kindness to us.

4. **Improve upon the worst.** Businesspeople always look at a problem by projecting the worst possible scenario. Then they put their energy into ensuring that the worst won't happen. We can often improve the end result if we take positive steps to prevent the most negative results.

5. **Be done with it.** Give the problem to God, with thanksgiving, and know that He can handle any situation. Then put the worry behind you; you've done all you can to take care of the problem. Refuse to allow it to continue bothering you. Declare that it is in the

hands of the King of kings and Lord of lords! When the cares try to reassert themselves, cast them on the Father afresh. Believe again in His sovereignty; apply His faithfulness to the details of life that seem to lure you into worry. Call on your Jehovah Jireh—"The Lord will provide."

In paintings artists use the method of perspective to portray different views of the same object. As Christians there is only one perspective we must have—the perspective of *eternity*. That perspective sets the tone for our lives. All our daily actions can be carried out against the background of eternity. Every decision, every action, every thought, every attitude is based on our eternal life through Christ. We're engulfed by Him and our lives are entwined with Him forever. Meditating on this spiritual reality will help us more deeply appreciate our Savior and Lord. As we humbly bow before Him in expressing our love and adoration for His sovereign care for our souls, we will be overwhelmed with His love and peace. In His strength we can face all of life's challenges without fear or worry.

DISCUSSION 🌿 QUESTIONS

1. What material goods do you value? Do you think of them as earthly treasures? Why or why not?

....

....

....

....

2. What are treasures in heaven? Do you think of yourself as having them? List ways this affects your daily life.

....

....

....

....

3. Each of us has a weakness for some material possession or circumstance. What's yours? How does Satan use it to make you worry?

....

....

....

....

4. Apply the five steps of analyzing worry to one current concern in your life. How does it help?

....

....

....

CHAPTER 6

WHO'S
IN CHARGE?

E ARTHQUAKES, TSUNAMIS, HURRICANES, wars, famines, and other large-scale tragedies strike millions of people in our world on a regular basis, making them feel helpless in the face of devastating loss. Despite our best efforts and knowledge and abilities, there are some events and circumstances over which we have no control. We can't control the stock market, which dictates how well our money might perform. We can't control another person's thoughts and feelings, which dictate how strong our relationships might be. And even if we eat right and exercise regularly, we can't completely control our physical well-being. Accidents, disease, and illness still happen.

Historian Barbara Tuchman said, "War is the unfolding of miscalculations."[1] Much of what goes on between nations is based upon a struggle for control. When a nation believes it can control another, or when a government thinks it can control its citizens, it miscalculates, and wars ensue.

On a personal level miscalculations can be just as chaotic or devastating as the events that shake our world. When we act as though we understand and can control events, circumstances, or people, we make a huge mistake. Manipulative control is another form of selfishness. Trying to control situations or people shows that we've replaced our trust in God with faith in ourselves to bring a desired outcome. But that kind of misplaced faith always results in failure.

Have you ever spent time with a two-year-old? Some of two-year-olds' favorite phrases are "mine," "no," and "I do it." They want to be independent. They think they know what they're doing. They have faith in their developing skills and abilities and judgment. Sometimes that streak of independence is frustrating to parents who have to wait as the child struggles to climb in and out of a car seat by himself. Sometimes it is dangerous. No matter how smart or capable a two-year-old is, he should not play with the stove or try to cross the street by himself.

But children persist in testing the limits of their independence. For instance, there's the little one who uses the kitchen drawers like a ladder to climb up to the counter. Like a kitten caught up in a tree, he gets stuck in a situation he's not equipped to handle. And only then does he start to worry about how he'll get down. Then comes the cry for help.

How often are we like that with God? Have you ever wanted to do it yourself rather than wait for Him? What happened? I think all of us are tempted to rely on our own brains and brawn. When we put our faith in ourselves, we lose sight of God's love and care. We're like that two-year-old climbing onto the kitchen counter. Once we get stuck, we get scared.

In order to know the personal presence of God in our lives, we must recognize the sovereign power of God as our Creator-Redeemer. If we are to find our purpose in His kingdom, we must give Him His rightful place as absolute sovereign deity. God's *sovereignty* speaks of His ruling over all as an all-wise King—benevolent, gracious, majestic, and powerful: "Our God is in heaven; he does whatever pleases him" (Ps. 115:3). God is love (1 John. 4:8). So we know it "pleases" Him to do good to His creation. That knowledge of God's sovereignty should motivate us to seek intimate relationship with our Creator, Lord, and Savior. As we receive that work of the Holy Spirit in our hearts, it will result in our experiencing the divine rest in His redemption for which we are ordained.

God declared His sovereignty through the prophet Isaiah (see Isaiah 46:9–10), and He reveals His sovereignty through His providential guidance and care. The Scriptures reveal His guiding hand throughout the history of mankind, and modern history corroborates the kindness of His providence. During wartime, soldiers have experienced inexplicable rescues and supernatural aid that only a loving God could accomplish. Testimonies of divine intervention in the lives of children, miraculous cures, and protection from natural disasters—all these things testify to the goodness of God's providential care.

When we integrate the reality of God's sovereignty into our faith, We will recognize that His grace is manifest in our lives. As we focus on His grace—His divine favor to us as created beings—we will be led to seek His provision for our salvation through His Son, Jesus Christ. When this happens, we begin to appreciate God as our Father, Redeemer, Provider, and Friend. All things exist because of the sovereign power of God. Our only response to this revelation is to bow in adoration and worship before Him. What a consolation to know that a power greater than ourselves can restore us to health and wholeness that God intended us to enjoy!

God's desire to keep us safe comes directly from His heart of love. Just as a faithful shepherd watches diligently over his sheep, the Lord, our Shepherd, delights in caring for us. Not only that, He's told us that He will eternally provide—in this world and the next. He wants us to trust Him to provide. However, when we're content to live selfishly, we care deeply about how much of worldly goods we obtain, and we try to control our possessions even as we calculate ways to get more. Yet those who trust in God don't care whether they have more or less. They know He will provide for them regardless.

> Trust in the LORD with all your heart, and lean not on your own understanding; in all your ways acknowledge Him, and He shall direct your paths.
> —PROVERBS 3:5–6, NKJV

A life of trust in God means we let Him guide us daily into His purposes. We hand Him our independence and our desire for control and let Him take the reins of our lives in His hands. This kind of trust-based lifestyle is not always easy. We can quickly grow comfortable with the beliefs and values of the world, even if we're filled with worry, falling into the habit of trusting ourselves and not trusting God. If we are to break this cycle, we must let go of worldly attitudes and firmly grasp God's hand, acknowledging His great faithfulness to us as well as His divine sovereignty in our lives. Then we can look for Him to lead us, acknowledging His control of our lives as we walk in trust and thanksgiving.

> When I am afraid, I put my trust in you. In God, whose word I praise—in God I trust and am not afraid. What can mere mortals do to me?
>
> —PSALM 56:3–4

I memorized this passage years ago. It helps me align myself with God and His Word, reminding me that God is in control and that I don't need to be afraid or try to be in charge myself. Reciting these verses in times of trouble has helped me worry less and trust more. God's Word can help you too.

DISCUSSION ✦ QUESTIONS

1. What circumstances beyond your control do you worry about? How can you release your desire for control?

....

....

....

2. When are you selfish? When are you reluctant to trust in God's ability to provide?

....

....

....

3. List some reasons that you can trust God.

....

....

....

4. Memorize Psalm 56:3–4 this week. Then recite these verses the next time you need encouragement about God's provision. List here how the verses helped.

....

....

....

....

CHAPTER 7

PEACE IN
GOD'S PROMISES

'M GETTING GRAY-HAIRED from worrying."

"Why are you worried?"

"Because I'm getting gray hair."

This fictitious conversation about worry might sound trite, but it shows the destructive cycle worry creates in our thinking. Once we start to worry about one area of our lives, it becomes easier to worry about another, and soon all we do is worry. Some patients I see are always worrying. I can offer many reassurances and give them all the information they need, yet they still worry. They're in the habit of worrying—about their cataract surgery, about their cars, about everything you could imagine. These folks' first reaction to a problem is worry.

Any of us could let worry become a way of thinking and a way of life. Worry produces negative thoughts that quickly lead to anxiety and fear. And negative thoughts produce negative people. I've been around negative people in my life, and I don't like it. I'm sure you've been around them too. Negative people constantly complain and criticize. Nothing is ever good enough for them.

When worry over a situation tries to set in, we need to challenge ourselves to respond in faith, not fear. The best way to replace that bad habit of worry is to create a good habit—looking to God's promises rather than our own feeble, human solutions. These promises are found in Scripture, which is God's own words. In His Word, He reminds us that He will intervene, He will help us, He will give fresh courage and strength. God will calm every storm in our lives as we trust Him

Throughout the Bible, God promises to provide for us. We should have no doubts, no fears, and no worries. We must remember God's pledges and promises to provide, especially in those times when we're tempted to worry rather than trust in His faithfulness.

> Taste and see that the LORD is good; blessed is the one who takes refuge in him. Fear the LORD, you his holy people, for those who fear him lack nothing. The lions may grow weak and hungry, but those who seek the LORD lack no good thing.
> —PSALM 34:8–10

THE BLAME GAME

Chronic worriers tend to quit taking responsibility for their actions at some point. As children they say, "My mother won't let me do this or that," or "The school won't let me do this." As they mature, they continue to find external reasons for their problems, believing the lie that they have no control over the events in their lives, but that other people do. They act as if they are pawns or victims. Instead of looking to God as the solution to all their problems, they blame others. For these people, it is always someone else's fault.

Breaking this destructive cycle begins by receiving an awareness that God loves us and will provide for us. The next step is to learn to live a life of surrender to God, having faith in His eternal promises and grace. His Word tells us that nothing can conquer those who truly believe in Him. His Word shows us the life of peace and joy Christ has provided for us through His redemption. As we allow faith in God's Word to fill our minds and hearts, destructive attitudes will be replaced by hope and trust in Him.

God has given us the ability to take responsibility for our actions and our lives. We must receive His promises and believe that we have the freedom to make positive choices that will benefit us to His glory. Blame looks to the past, which can't be changed. Responsibility looks to the future, which can be taken care of and managed through the grace of God.

DO WE MEASURE UP?

There are times in each of our lives when we compare ourselves with others. We might get jealous of the new car our neighbor buys or when someone else in the company gets the promotion we think we should have gotten. We might even wonder whether our children are as successful as the children of our friends.

Jesus talks about this attitude in the parable of the prodigal son. Most of the story is about the younger son, who demanded his inheritance from his father and wasted it. However, when the younger son "came to himself" and decided to return home, his father welcomed him with open arms and threw a huge party. When the older son, who had stayed at home and worked faithfully for his father, heard about the party, he was furious. He thought it was unfair that his father should be so generous to a son that the older son judged as undeserving.

But his father was not concerned with *fair*; he was revealing the loving heart of a father for a lost son. He spoke to his older son.

> My son…you are always with me, and everything I have is yours. But we had to celebrate and be glad, because this brother of yours was dead and is alive again; he was lost and is found.
>
> —Luke 15:31–32

The father had a greater vision. He loved both of his sons and rejoiced in their well-being. That is the heart of God. As much as we might worry or complain about whether we measure up to another's success, we need to remember that God does not compare us with others; He loves each of us as His children.

FEAR OF MAN OR LOVE OF GOD

Another life situation that causes some to worry is whether people like and accept them and on what basis.

As I grew up, I saw young girls whose parents didn't accept them.

They had no peace. With hearts in turmoil from this rejection, they sought acceptance in all the wrong ways. Some worked out their sexuality in ways that cost them satisfaction in their lives. Rather than the acceptance they sought, their behavior brought much pain upon themselves and others. Instead of seeking to know God's great love and receive His acceptance, they tried to find acceptance in their efforts that created more emotional pain in the end.

There is nothing as great as God's eternal love, given to us to receive by His grace. In His unfathomable goodness, He desires that we, His children, experience total well-being of body, mind, and spirit. God knows that nothing can satisfy our hearts like His abiding presence in our lives, and He wants us to know it too. God's great love satisfies our hearts and gives us purpose in life.

When we dare to take our eyes off people to find acceptance we long for and turn to God, we can be freed from those destructive forces that grip our lives. Not only does the grace of God bring salvation to our hearts (Eph. 2:8), it also keeps us in the love of God, protecting us from destructive forces. The apostle Paul learned to say: "By the grace of God I am what I am" (1 Cor. 15:10). It is not the acceptance of people that should affect our lives fundamentally. It is what God says about us as He shows us His great love and acceptance in His Word that we should value and believe.

The innate desire for acceptance is strong in human nature. If we don't embrace the grace of God's acceptance of us in Christ, we can act out in many ways to seek acceptance from others. The drive to find acceptance and the frustration of not finding it may cause us to live recklessly. We may be reckless in the way we drive a car or run a business or spend money. We may become belligerent, aggressive, or violent, trying to earn others' acceptance and respect. We may be sexually irresponsible, seeking a false sense of security and love. All these behaviors indicate that we are more worried about the acceptance, or lack of it, from people than our acceptance from God, whose love for us is eternal.

We need to get back in the good habit of practicing faith in God and remembering His grace. If God accepts us as believing sinners through the cross of Christ, and if He will provide everything we need, why should we be worried about what others think and do. If as believers we're busy worrying about what others think of us, we become selfish, and our wills are no longer aligned with the will of God.

In this pitiful state our relationship with the Lord declines. We lose the closeness and the rest and peace He gives us. Instead, we feel like we do in a relationship with a person with whom we were once close but are now distant from. We can't really talk to them; there's no emotional intimacy anymore. How does this pitiful state of being come about? It can begin very simply by taking our eyes off our relationship with God and instead becoming critical or envious of others, worrying about what they think and how we compare with them.

Climbing out of that hole begins when we determine to fill our minds with God's Word and spend time in His presence. When we decide that what God says about us is more important than how we measure up in people's eyes, we realize that there is nothing as important as God and our relationship with Him. This eternal perspective helps us live with freedom and peace and joy; it sets us free from worry and helps us not to be critical and judgmental of others.

FEAR OF LONELINESS

Because we are created in the image of God, each of us has an innate, inner longing for relationship with the eternal God, of which we may not be aware. When that longing is not satisfied by the grace we receive from God through the Holy Spirit, we become lonely. Our hearts are seeking something, and the many possessions and jobs and relationships we have tried don't seem to fill the void. Sometimes we believe if we just rush around enough, keep busy enough, and surround ourselves with enough important and interesting people, our loneliness will disappear.

"Loneliness and the feeling of being unwanted is the most terrible poverty," Mother Teresa said.[1] We often fear this loneliness, and we try to ignore it by manipulating others to get love and attention from them. Or we try to fill the void by seeking people as possessions, not as genuine relationships. This fear is very dangerous. It causes many people to make bad choices regarding friends and marriage partners, resulting in harmful relationships and wrong marriages.

The Bible doesn't simply say that God *loves* or that He *has* love; it states plainly: "God *is* love" (1 John 4:8, emphasis added). We were created by love. Is it any wonder that the human heart craves love so deeply and on so many levels? We were made by love—to walk in relationship with God, who is love. Blaise Pascal, a seventeenth-century French physicist and philosopher, wrote:

> There is a God-shaped vacuum in the heart of each man which cannot be satisfied by any created thing, but only by God the Creator, made known through Jesus Christ.[2]

Learning to appreciate God's presence in our lives by receiving Christ as our Savior is imperative if we are to satisfy our deepest desire for love. We can live emotionally fulfilled lives only when we give ourselves to Christ in a personal love relationship He made possible for us at Calvary. Personal relationship with Christ changes who we are and how we relate to others. Knowing the love of God personally helps us to make divine connections with others through the Holy Spirit. Such godly friendships are selective, sacrificial, steadfast, and secure—totally committed, when each person is willing to do anything for the other. These kinds of friendships lead us out of loneliness as God works to make our lives more meaningful.

THE LURE OF MONEY

If we are honest, most of us frequently worry about money. We tend to live in awe of it, viewing it as the world's measuring stick of accomplishments because the world tells us that we will succeed and gain respect if we earn enough money. In this temporal, worldly perspective, all of life is evaluated by money—money status, money power, money obtained from work, money needed, the fear of not having enough money in the future, and the fear of losing the money presently in hand. Oftentimes we think more about money than we think about God.

This kind of thinking can have us worshipping money with no time left to worship God. When this happens, money has displaced God in our lives. In fact it can become our god. Many people who are very interested in the Lord are lured by the love of money. Focusing on money more than God inevitably leads to more worry and less peace.

There is a deceitfulness to riches that says money promises everything. In reality, money appears to give some things, but actually gives nothing of eternal value. True satisfaction cannot be purchased with any amount of money. Anyone who has wrestled with this issue knows that the fear of losing money or running out of money can be worse than the reality if that happened.

When we worry that we won't have enough money to meet our needs, we are not trusting God's promises to supply all our needs. We are forgetting His eternal perspective and allowing our worry to control us.

This inordinate fear of not having enough money ages us, altars our good judgment, and can eventually consume and control our lives, taking our focus off of the love of God and His promises to meet all our needs. The mind games we play show that we are devious in our pursuit of money and not devoted to God. For example, how can we worship God on Sunday and cheat on our taxes—or anything else— throughout the week? We fool ourselves if we think finances are of such great importance that we must be dishonest in our financial dealings.

Money is not worth cheating to obtain. Our true worth is not measured by having money in the bank or acquiring many possessions. Our inestimable value was measured on the cross, where Christ died to redeem us and to give us true riches of eternal life. Our true worth is reflected by our response in faith and thanksgiving to Jesus for His death and resurrection. Our true sustenance is the presence of Jesus in our lives. Jesus taught: "Watch out! Be on your guard against all kinds of greed; life does not consist in an abundance of possessions" (Luke 12:15).

COUNTING THE COST

Here's an exercise you can try. If you start getting too worried or anxious about a situation, take a step back from it. You might even try walking up to a mirror, looking yourself in the eye, and asking the question "Is this worth the devastating effects that worry will have on my well-being?" Jesus answered that question for us.

> Are not five sparrows sold for two pennies? Yet not one of them is forgotten by God. Indeed, the very hairs of your head are all numbered. Don't be afraid; you are worth more than many sparrows.
>
> —LUKE 12:6–7

God loves us and treasures us as His children. He has everything under control for all eternity. All we need to do is remember to look to Him and let Him provide all He has promised in His Word. Praise be to God for His infinite wisdom and mercy! Amen.

DISCUSSION 🌿QUESTIONS

1. Do you know someone who plays "the blame game"? How can knowing 2 Corinthians 4:8–10 help?

2. When have you compared yourself with others? How does it help you? How does it hurt you?

3. When have you felt lonely? What helps you out of that feeling?

4. What helps you find meaningful relationships with others?

5. How important is money to you? Do you think you have enough? What does God say about how much is enough?

CHAPTER 8

DIVINE WEAPONS
AGAINST WORRY

ORRY AND FEAR take root in our lives when our selfish interest keeps us from being aligned with God's eternal purposes. This happens because we do not embrace His perspective of life, for the present or for the future. Instead, we get tangled up in our own material, earthly concerns and worry about how we will make it all happen. We start fearing events and circumstances beyond our control until chronic worry begins to destroy us. In our worried state we can't think straight, can't sort out our emotions. We act irrationally, making poor decisions. All of this can put us into a serious state of physical and mental stress that can eventually kill us if left unchecked.

Before you get into such a pitiful state, you need to ask yourself some very important questions. What worries you? What is putting a brake on your physical, emotional, and spiritual health? How long has this been going on? Can you release that brake? Can you get rid of the worry? Can you get rid of the selfishness?

The answer to all these questions comes down to one thing: when we surrender our lives to God, He gives us victory. He gives all believers victory over all sin—including selfishness and worry—through the person of Jesus Christ! Jesus understands our human nature, and He has the answer to every worry, every fear, every problem. He knows that the worry and fear we experience are worse than the actual situation that precipitates our fear. For example, it is worse for our well-being to worry about being hungry than to actually be hungry; it is worse to worry about having enough money to buy the right clothes, worse to worry about being able to live the lifestyle we want to live.

Jesus knows that worry destroys the beautiful peace and rest in His redemption that He died to give us. He came to rescue us from worry and fear in making it possible for God to live within us, reconciling us to His divine peace. The basic treatment for worry is to live a life of thanksgiving for God's grace we receive in His salvation—eternal life and His divine provision for this earthly life, all bought for us on the cross of Jesus' sacrifice.

When we truly open our hearts to our Redeemer, we discover such love and peace that all we can do is bow before Him in humble adoration and worship for His loving care. We begin to value His presence in our lives more than anything else. And we can walk up the gangplank of faith, full of thanksgiving, into the ship of God's grace, trusting in His divine favor to meet the needs of every situation in life that we face.

When we are tempted to fear difficult challenges in life or worry about any situation that confronts us, we can use the divine weapons Christ has given us to defeat these enemies of our soul. Let's look more deeply into the weapons of faith, grace, and thanksgiving, through Christ, that can help us defeat worry and fear.

FAITH

There is a story about a fellow from the country who, after years of avoiding flying out of fear, had to make his first airplane trip. The trip was uneventful; he reached his destination and returned home safely. Upon his return, a friend asked him how he handled his fear of flying. "Well, to tell you the truth," he said, "I never did put all my weight down on the airplane."

Have you ever done that? There have been times in my own life when I've been reluctant to "put all my weight down" on Christ. I was just not quite sure I had faith for Him to help me through a tough time or predicament. Then the inevitable happened. The situation got far worse. I should have trusted in the Lord in the first place instead of putting my weight on my own shoulders. Trusting ourselves is the opposite of what God wants us to do. He asks us to place our trust and confidence in His sovereign power and perfect love. He promises He will take care of us; we don't need to worry.

What beautiful promises are found in Psalm 21! "The king shall have joy in Your strength, O LORD.... You have given him his heart's desire, and have not withheld the request of his lips.... He asked life from You, and You gave it to him—length of days forever and ever.... Be exalted, O LORD, in Your own strength! We will sing and praise Your power" (vv. 1–2, 4, 13, NKJV). As any good earthly father watches over a child, so God watches over His children. We can rest our entire weight on Him; we can place all our faith in Him. Then our minds will be at peace, and we will learn to rest in His wonderful redemption. His love alone can satisfy our hearts and set us free from fear and worry.

Faith functions in our lives in almost unconscious ways. Take the law of gravity, for instance. As adults our actions are subjected to an understanding of the power of the gravitational force under which we function. When we go into an exclusive shop where fine china or other exquisite glass creations are sold, we are very careful not to drop a vase or any other breakable. We know that the law of gravity is working and that such an accident would result in breaking valuable merchandise because we have explicit faith in the law of gravity. God wants us to have this same kind of explicit faith in Him. He is the Creator of all that exists around us.

In 1692 Isaac Newton wrote, "So then Gravity may put the Planets into Motion, but without the divine Power it could never put them into such a circulating motion as they have about the sun; and therefore, for this, as well as other Reasons, I am compelled to ascribe the Frame of the System to an intelligent Agent.... The Cause of Gravity is what I do not pretend to know."[1] Dr. Richard Swenson writes that "although Sir Isaac Newton clarified the law of gravity several hundred years ago, it remains a mysterious force.... If we drop a pencil, it falls to the floor. Why?... At the deepest level, we don't know. Yet if God were to suspend the law of gravity, we would need a steel cable six hundred miles in diameter to hold the moon in place."[2]

As we pause to consider scientific phenomena such as the mystery of the law of gravity, the wonder of creation will transcend our finiteness and help us place our faith in this sovereign God, who is love (1 John 4:8). Though such an infinite Creator God must inevitably remain mysterious to our finite minds, as we place our faith in Him, we can acknowledge His power and surrender all things, including our worry and fear, to His infinite love.

There's one biblical account of profound faith in God that always speaks to me. It's the story from Genesis chapter 22 of Abraham, father of Isaac who was willing to sacrifice what he loved most because he trusted in God. You may remember that Isaac's birth was miraculous, being conceived after Sarah and Abraham were too old to have children.

How they must have rejoiced in the miraculous birth of this son. Then, when Isaac was a young man, God tells Abraham to take him, this heir of promise, to the land of Moriah and sacrifice him as a burnt offering. No loving father would want to sacrifice his son. Abraham and Sarah had waited so long to have Isaac. How could Abraham yield to God's command to give him up? What would he tell Sarah? Everything about this command from God seemed contrary to the promise God had made to Abraham that "it is through Isaac that your offspring will be reckoned" (Gen. 21:12).

Yet in faith Abraham prepared to obey His God, placing all his faith in Him. He collected the wood for the burnt offering, packed up his donkey, and headed off with Isaac. When they got close to Mount Moriah, Isaac became curious, wanting to know where the lamb was for the burnt offering. "God himself will provide the lamb," Abraham said (Gen. 22:8), showing total trust in the God he had followed and trusted with his life. When they got to the place where God had told him to sacrifice his son, Abraham began preparing for the sacrifice. He built the altar, arranged the wood, and then he tied up Isaac and put him on top of the wood. Finally he pulled out his knife to kill his son. At that very moment, the angel of the Lord called out to him.

"Do not lay a hand on the boy," he said. "Do not do anything
to him. Now I know that you fear God, because you have not
withheld from me your son, your only son."

—GENESIS 22:12

It was then that Abraham saw a ram caught in some bushes.
Understanding that the ram was God's provision for the sacrifice He
had commanded, Abraham sacrificed it on that altar in place of his
son. "To this day it is said, 'On the mountain of the LORD it will be provided'" (Gen. 22:14). A new name was given to this place to encourage
all believers to cheerfully trust wholly in God's goodness: Jehovah
Jireh, "the Lord will provide." Was Abraham worried? Scripture does
not say that he was. His actions seem to indicate immediate obedience
because of his faith in God. Faith was his great weapon against worry
and fear in the face of losing his promised heir.

Abraham's encounter gives me faith because it helps me remember
that God, as our Father and our Shepherd, will always provide in our
greatest time of trial. I believe He is intimately involved in my daily life.
This "knowing" is not just in my head but in my heart, and it leads me
continually into a deeper life of faith.

I have been crucified with Christ and I no longer live, but
Christ lives in me. The life I now live in the body, I live by
faith in the Son of God, who loved me and gave himself for
me.

—GALATIANS 2:20

Living a life of faith means living fully surrendered to Christ in the
kingdom of God. When we live fully in His kingdom, we focus on God
in all the moments of our days, thankful for His love and His work
in our lives, expressing our appreciation and thankfulness to Him.
Prayerfully we do our planning to execute His will in our lives, laying
the groundwork, acting responsibly, and trusting God for the results.

Scripture teaches us that faith is a gift of God to us and not something we can manufacture. This gift has many facets. For example,
there is the gift of faith that brings us to salvation through Christ (Eph.
2:8–9). After receiving this salvation gift, we must seek to grow in our

faith through reading the Scriptures, praying, and exercising our faith to uproot the unbelief in our minds. This unbelief often manifests itself as thoughts of fear and worry and lack of trust in our Lord's faithfulness and sovereignty. As we read the Scriptures, we learn to appreciate God's love and faithfulness toward us, and we begin to be filled with faith in Him. That faith is expressed through praise and thanksgiving, worship and adoration. Pursuing growth in faith is vitally important if we want to please God.

> And without faith it is impossible to please God, because anyone who comes to him must believe that he exists and that he rewards those who earnestly seek him.
>
> —HEBREWS 11:6

Faith is also the essence of our strength in the eternal God. When we have this kind of strengthening faith in the person of Jesus Christ, the godly characteristics of joy, peace, and hope can blossom forth from our lives. George Mueller once said it this way: "Where faith begins, anxiety ends; for where anxiety begins, faith ends."[3] Our faith in Christ is a powerful weapon to oust every vestige of fear and worry from our minds and hearts.

Life continually hits us with waves of good events and bad circumstances. These life events can create anxiety or joy, happiness or fear. Satan would love to use those bad times to undermine our faith in God. He would love for us to give in to our fears and anxieties and to forget God's loving promises of provision, choosing rather to rely on our weak human efforts.

But our weapon of faith says we're content in our present state; it says we have enough, whether we are rich or poor, healthy or sick, young or old. Regardless of temporal circumstances and events, we know our daily strength comes from the Lord. The only real security and stability we have in this life is found in our faith in Jesus Christ. With Jesus we can stand firm in faith, knowing God provides all we need to face every situation in life, good or bad.

Paul, who was imprisoned many times, demonstrated through his faith in Christ that we can be happy and content regardless of our circumstances when we have faith in Christ. Locked in prison, Paul still rejoiced because his joy was in Christ, not dependent on external circumstances. (See Philippians 4:11–12.) What a testimony of faith! Like Abraham, Paul knew the Lord as his Jehovah Jireh—his provider. He saw the circumstances in his life from an eternal perspective. He had an unshakable assurance of faith in the person of Jesus Christ. And he knew the abundance of God's grace—that God loved him so much He would always sustain him.

Paul and Abraham are giants of the faith who show us that we don't need to be afraid. When our "treasure" is with God and our faith is in Him, this world can do nothing to truly harm us. We can live in peace and rest in His redemption by our knowledge of and belief in eternal life in the person of Jesus Christ. Our faith rests in knowing that we belong to the Creator, Redeemer, and Sustainer of the universe. We are His children, and He will protect us and provide for us. We have nothing to fear because the Lord will take care of us now and for eternity. We will delve more deeply into the power of living a life of courageous faith in Chapter 10.

GRACE

The Scriptures define *grace* simply as God's favor, His undeserved kindness bestowed on our lives. When we receive salvation through Christ, we are receiving the redeeming grace of God and enjoying His divine favor on our lives. The apostle Paul declared of himself: "But by the grace of God I am what I am" (1 Cor. 15:10). By the grace of God we are what we are. It is by God's divine favor that we receive in accepting Christ as our Savior that we are redeemed, reconciled to God. Everything we receive from God is accomplished by the grace of God. We just have to get it through our heads, our hearts, our pride, and our own sense of self-importance that by receiving God's grace, we allow Him to love us and provide for us beyond our understanding.

Why does God love such selfish, rebellious, independent people as you and me? Why does He love us even though we worry and fret and complain? Certainly not because we deserve it. He loves us because of His grace—His divine favor.

> For it is by grace you have been saved, through faith—and this is not from yourselves, it is the gift of God—not by works, so that no one can boast.
>
> —EPHESIANS 2:8–9

Our actions and accomplishments do not save us. Trusting in the person of Christ and the salvation His death on the cross wrought for us is what saves us. If we were treated *fairly*—given what we *deserved*—none of us would be spending eternity with our Creator, Redeemer, and Sustainer. This is a humbling truth. That is why we must humble ourselves in order to place our faith in Christ and forgiveness and His grace.

As we humble our hearts to admit our need of God, He manifests to us His grace and love and gives us His divine presence to dwell in our hearts. Then our hearts are filled with awe and gratitude for this loving God, who forgives our sin and gives us His peace and all we need for life. His divine love satisfies every longing of our hearts and causes us to bow in worship before His throne of grace and to express our deep appreciation of who He is and what He has done for us.

When grace is present, we surrender to His will and feel the profound security of His firm fingers of control over our lives. Embraced by God in this divine grace, we discover that it is a weapon against worry and fear. Then we are filled with joy because we know we're protected by His love and will live with Him forever. This realization of the eternal power of the resurrection life of Christ within us is ours for eternity.

God's Word reassures us of His promises and strengthens our belief in His grace, which is sufficient not only now but for eternity because we are *His* forever and His provision is forever. We're intertwined and engulfed in His love forever. When we realize the beauty of God's future grace to take care of us for all eternity, we can understand the purpose of creation and that our purpose in living is to rest in His redemption and enjoy intimate relationship with Him—eternally.

THANKSGIVING

Banks Anderson, a professor emeritus of ophthalmology at Duke, was once asked, "If you had only one choice of medicine for a health condition, what would you take?" He said, "Corticosteroids, of course. They can treat many ophthalmologic diseases; more than any other medicine" because they can knock down inflammation. They can treat more diseases than any antibiotic or immunosuppressant agent.

When you ask me what I consider to be the best therapy for worry, I will tell you unequivocally that a thankful heart, as we discussed, is the "corticosteroid" for worry. The apostle Paul tells us how powerful a weapon thanksgiving is for our well-being.

> Rejoice in the Lord always. I will say it again: Rejoice! Let your gentleness be evident to all. The Lord is near. Do not be anxious about anything, but in every situation, by prayer and petition, with thanksgiving, present your requests to God. And the peace of God, which transcends all understanding, will guard your hearts and your minds in Christ Jesus.
> —PHILIPPIANS 4:4–7

Paul is talking about creating a habit and living a lifestyle of thanksgiving—he is describing a thanksgiving frenzy, if you will. What is a thanksgiving frenzy? I define it as an intense lifestyle, a lavish expression of thanksgiving, a mental attitude of continual thanks to God that permeates every thought, defining our relationship with God and impacting our relationship with others and even our approach to our vocation. If we are to experience an intimate relationship with our eternal God, we must be thankful to Him from the depths of our being.

To be thankful to Him means to give thanks in all things. This kind of thankfulness cultivates a spirit of thanksgiving in our hearts until we overflow with profound gratitude for the person of Jesus Christ living in us. We become thankful for the grace that saves us, the grace that forgives our sin and accepts our repentance. Being thankful helps us realize who God is and who we are as His beloved children. This heightened awareness of our Creator causes us to stand in gratitude because of His continual forgiveness of our sins and of rebellion against Him. Indeed, we cannot truly give heartfelt thanks until we realize that we are nothing on our own yet everything through Him.

When our hearts overflow with praise in the knowledge of who God is, we can't help but express our wonder and awe for His eternal love in our lives; we reverently worship and adore Him as our sovereign, loving Lord. This profound life of thanksgiving and praise is a powerful weapon to quench any temptation to fear or worry. Hearts full of praise and worship are healthy hearts that have hope for the present and the future. We are His for all eternity! What joy!

Through personal experience I have come to believe that thankfulness is a nonnegotiable priority of the life of every believer. Some of us say the words "thank you" so often that they become a part of us. Others are quiet and express "thank you" with a touch, a look, an attitude of care and concern—understanding and appreciating without words. We're all different, and rightfully so. But each of us must express our spirit of thanksgiving to God in a meaningful way.

Luke describes how one man demonstrated the thankful spirit in chapter 17 of his Gospel. Ten men were healed by Jesus, but only one man came back to Jesus in thanksgiving. Only one related to Him personally in expressing gratitude for the gift of healing he had received. This one man exemplifies the thankful heart each of us should have toward God. When we are focused on God in the person of Jesus Christ, we're thankful for everything we have.

A thankful spirit not only is reflected in our relationship with God but extends to our relationships with our loved ones and friends, strengthening them out of our gratitude. For example, in marriage our steadfast thankfulness produces strength, support, and growth in our love for each other. Our continual gestures of thankfulness, love, and affirming support give our spouse a sense of self-worth as we build a deeper relationship of trust and love. In the same way, we need to be thankful for friends, family, and coworkers—all those with whom we rub shoulders in our daily lives. We can serve, we can give, we can be partners, and we can love others when we have a genuine spirit of thanksgiving for others.

The spirit of thankfulness must be woven into the fabric of everything we, as followers of Christ, do. In every activity, whether it's performing delicate surgery, writing books, presenting a legal defense, or sweeping a hall, we should have an attitude of gratitude that springs from a thankful heart for God's loving care for us.

Being thankful establishes our faith to rest in His grace. This brief discussion of our divine weapons of faith, grace, and thanksgiving, springing from our relationship with the person of Jesus Christ, shows us how to rid our lives of worry and fear. These weapons allow our lives to be engulfed by the presence of God—now and for eternity. That profound relationship with our Savior is the ultimate antidote for worry!

DISCUSSION ⚘ QUESTIONS

1. What does *faith* mean to you? How do you see faith at work in your daily life?

....

....

....

....

2. What does *grace* mean to you? List some ways you sense God's grace.

....

....

....

....

3. What does *thanksgiving* mean to you? When do you feel most thankful? Least thankful? List five ways you can be more thankful. Practice at least one way every day this week.

....

....

....

4. Try having a good laugh first thing in the morning. Does it change your outlook on the day?

....

....

....

....

CHAPTER 9

SUPERNATURAL BIRTH
INTO THE KINGDOM OF GOD

A T THE BATTLE of the Alamo, Colonel William B. Travis asked his men to cross the line to give themselves in defending the provisional government in San Antonio as it sought Texas' independence from Mexico. That call came at great personal cost. All two hundred defenders died at the Alamo.[1] That battle was a turning point in American history.

Similarly, when we accept Christ as our Savior and are born again into the kingdom of God, Christ asks all of us to cross the line—to abandon ourselves to His eternal purposes. He asks us to put aside our own agendas and desires and to submit our lives totally to Him. We are not first called to *do works* for Him, but to *surrender* to the lordship of Christ. That act of obedience to our Lord implies denying ourselves and placing our faith and trust in His grace to save us and to order our lives according to His eternal purposes. As those brave warriors at the Alamo determined to obey the command of their leader, each of us faces a personal turning point in our lives when we surrender to the lordship of Christ.

Receiving His forgiveness for our sins and the promise of His presence dwelling within us for eternity, He becomes our Lord and Master. We cannot continue to serve our earthly desires or goals any longer.

No one can serve two masters. Either you will hate the one and love the other, or you will be devoted to the one and despise the other. You cannot serve both God and Money.

—MATTHEW 6:24

When you think about all the advertisements on television, in magazines, and online for ways to live longer and look younger, you realize that people will do anything to preserve their natural life. Yet according to the Scriptures, there's only one way to truly preserve life for eternity, and that's found in the person of Jesus Christ. Life truly begins when we believe what Christ accomplished at Calvary for our redemption, giving us eternal life.

At the moment we accept Christ's provision for the forgiveness of our sins, we are no longer simply preserving our temporal lives; we are born into the kingdom of God and receive eternal life through Christ. The forgiveness of sins, the grace of God, and the hope of eternity with God all become ours at that moment we place our faith in our Savior. In an attitude of repentance we hand over the reins of our lives to His will and direction, admitting that we've been independent and rebellious. Turning from selfish, self-centered ways, we begin our journey to transformation into the image and character of Christ through trusting Him as our faithful and sovereign Lord and Savior.

Jesus says we must decide whom we are going to serve. In fact He demands that we make that choice. Do we say yes to Jesus Christ, who loves us and gave Himself as a sacrifice for our sins through His death on the cross in order that we could be reconciled to peace with God? That is not a decision to be taken lightly. Saying yes to Christ means making a total commitment that involves loving Him with our hearts, minds, souls, and strength, and expressing that love every day in faith and thanksgiving.

Paul describes this total commitment in Romans 12:1 as an act of worship: "Therefore, I urge you, brothers and sisters, in view of God's mercy, to offer your bodies as a living sacrifice, holy and pleasing to God—this is your true and proper worship." The Scriptures teach that worship is not merely an *external* expression of thanksgiving and praise to God; it is best expressed through complete *surrender* to His lordship over our lives.

Christianity is introduced to the world in the person of Jesus—the miracle of His birth, His life, His death on the cross to save us from our sins, and His amazing resurrection from the dead, which gives us eternal life and fellowship with Him. When we receive Christ as our Savior, we are born into the kingdom of God. What He asks of us in surrendering to His wonderful redemption is to change our earthly focus, to repent of our selfishness and worldly desires, and to embrace His transforming power in our lives to realize our eternal purpose. This change of focus demands that we humble ourselves in His presence in gratitude for His salvation and the gift of eternal life. Jesus demonstrated this attitude of humility during His time on earth in his complete obedience to His Father, even to death on the cross.

When we say yes to the person of Jesus Christ, completely and without reservation, the eternal kingdom of God is born in us, as I mentioned. As born-again believers the journey toward a life filled with joy begins as we surrender our lives wholeheartedly to God and become His children, cleansed and transformed by His love for all eternity. As we experience the satisfying presence of God in our lives through our surrender to Christ's lordship, we discover that He is the source of ultimate joy. He is the author of our peace, and in Him we find true rest and fulfillment for our souls.

When we are born into the kingdom of God, I have found there to be three vital elements on our journey to a joy-filled life. In addition to *faith* and *grace*, which we discussed earlier, there is the element of *relinquishment* to His love and His will that fills us with joy. When we truly appreciate God's grace, we cannot help but relinquish everything to Him in faith because of His goodness. As children in the kingdom of God our focus and values and pursuits can no longer be those of the world but of His kingdom. We begin to see life differently with our hearts filled with God's love. We no longer seek satisfaction and fulfillment in the things of this world because surrendering to God separates us from much of the thinking of the world. Instead, we begin to develop an eternal perspective—an ever-growing measure of satisfaction now and forever in God through the person of Jesus Christ.

As God's eternal kingdom begins to take hold in our lives, we no longer put our faith in the "goals" for happiness as the world perceives them to be, based on gratification of the immediate, the seen, and the now. Instead, we put our faith in God—eternal faith, based on the promise of Christ and our Father to provide for us now and forever. This is not faith based on a weak human emotion. Rather, it is faith focused on God's power, love, and grace that we received in salvation, being born into the kingdom of God. As we learn to trust His faithfulness and sovereign rule over all, our hearts are filled with great joy that leads to ever deeper worship and adoration as we bow in humility in the presence of our Lord.

Scripture teaches that this life is but a vapor, appearing for a little while and then vanishing (Jas. 4:14). Whatever age we are, we tend to feel the march of time militating against us. Many who are in their forties think the past twenty years have gone by too quickly. Those in their sixties think the past twenty years have gone even faster. However, when we live with God's eternal perspective, seeing Him as our Jehovah Jireh, we see time simply as the preamble to eternity. God's eternal perspective enables us to live secure in the knowledge that He will care for us now and for all eternity.

As a father I really haven't concerned myself much with my own circumstances and possessions, but I have always wanted to make sure my children were taken care of. Now that I'm a grandfather, I feel that desire even more for my grandchildren. I believe this is the same way the Father feels about us. He wants to make sure we're provided for in every way during this lifetime and beyond. And because He's God, He *can* meet all our needs—now and for eternity. As His beloved children, we can surrender our anxieties and fears, receive His provision, and live with hope and freedom. That was the purpose in Christ's ultimate sacrifice. "It is for freedom that Christ has set us free. Stand firm, then, and do not let yourselves be burdened again by a yoke of slavery" (Gal. 5:1).

All of us worry about one thing or another, and we can become slaves to our worry, as we discussed. It is God's grace that sets us free. He has taken responsibility for looking out for us. No matter how difficult life might seem today, when we surrender our lives to Christ, we can be thankful, for we are placed into His unshakable kingdom forever. Hebrews 12:28 says, "Therefore, since we are receiving a kingdom that cannot be shaken, let us be thankful."

Oftentimes when we are in the midst of life's challenges, thankfulness seems hard. Yet God is there to help us, providing the support we need in tough times. He will be our constant companion if we let Him. God, the author of the universe, promises He will abide with us in this process of surrender and transformation. "I can do all this through him who gives me strength" (Phil. 4:13). Our own strength is never sufficient. Our feeble, fallible, human efforts will fail, and we will fall victim to all forms of selfishness and worry, anxiety and fear, and pride and control. Only through our continual surrender to the lordship of Christ can we be transformed into His image: godliness, love, joy, and peace. We must be completely honest with ourselves and realize Christ is all and we are nothing. Our safety from destructive emotions and thought patterns is in that place of surrender to His lordship.

Unless the LORD builds the house, the builders labor in vain.
—PSALM 127:1

As believers who have received salvation through Christ, God has begun a work in us, and He will see it through. Jesus will perfect us; He will mature us; He will transform us. He will continue to work in our lives until we see Him face to face. In the midst of the process, we need to be able to say: "God, I thank You that You began a good work in me. I thank You that no matter how unfinished I am at the moment, You will gloriously complete Your work on the day of Christ Jesus. Heavenly Father, help me to cooperate with You as You mold me into the likeness of Jesus. Amen."

We say with Paul, "I can do all things through Christ who strengthens me" (Phil. 4:13, NKJV), because we have the spiritual strength of knowing that God's sovereign power has control over our lives for all eternity. We have faith in Christ to help us conquer fears, and we have exceeding gratitude for our redemption that will vanquish worries. We also have His peace and His power, enabling us in all areas of life.

...being confident of this, that he who began a good work in you will carry it on to completion until the day of Christ Jesus.

—PHILIPPIANS 1:6

In the next chapter let's look more deeply into the way we can live a courageous life of faith filled with God's wonderful grace.

DISCUSSION ❧ QUESTIONS

1. Have you crossed the line to commit your life to Jesus? If not, are you willing to do so now?

....

....

....

2. List some ways Jesus has changed you since you surrendered yourself to Him.

....

....

....

3. How much have you grasped of the three essential elements of your journey toward a life of joy: grace, relinquishment, and faith?

....

....

....

4. How do you sense Christ's presence in your life? How are you aware of His transforming power in your life now? Keep a journal this week recording the ways you realize His presence.

....

....

5. What steps do you need to take to fully rest, without fear, in the hands of Jesus?

....

....

CHAPTER 10

LIVING IN
COURAGEOUS FAITH

E ARLIER WE DISCUSSED the divine weapons God has given us to combat worry and fear: grace, faith, and thanksgiving. As we delve deeper into what a life of faith looks like, we will understand more fully how God calls all believers to live with courageous faith. What does that really mean? We know that when we are being reckless in making life decisions, it causes us to worry. Reckless investors worry. Reckless fantasies and reckless sexuality cause worry. Even reckless driving creates a tension of worry in our minds. Therefore, it's vital to our peace of mind that we choose to be careful in our decisions and our actions.

In reality, living life as Christian is the most conservative and safest lifestyle available to us. Surrendering to the will of God for our lives gives us a sense of security as we trust His love for us. Learning to rest in His redemption, we experience His joy and peace and the confidence He gives to us through His promise that He will never leave us or forsake us. When we love God, we are empowered by the Holy Spirit to reject the mindset of fear and worry and we realize we have adopted the safest lifestyle possible.

However, in our walk with God we will sometimes face challenges that require us to make decisions that seem to us to be a bit reckless. We will have to summon our faith and courage to obey God's will for us when we do not understand what He is asking, as in Abraham's life when he obeyed God's command to sacrifice his son, his heir of promise God had given to him.

When instructors teach skiing, they say, "You have to be a bit of a fool to be a good skier." When the instructor says to be a little foolish, he's not telling us to go and break a leg (as I've done). He's telling us to relax and muster the courage to take a chance. Without that element of "recklessness," we will never experience the truly great feeling of flying down that snowy slope. In other words, we can't be overly anxious or lacking in courage if we are to be a good skier.

So how does that analogy apply to life? What does it mean to live with courageous faith? It means freeing ourselves from anxious worries about every little life concern. A person who is free of the obsessions of worry is able to relax and do a good job, enjoying every area of life. When we're totally relaxed in skiing, we can employ a kind of courage called *anticipation*. That involves just relaxing and dropping down on the lower ski, which allows the rebound phenomenon to carry us into a turn on that challenging ski slope. It is almost effortless to do mid-turns smoothly as we get the *anticipation* technique down. The key is the more we relax, the more effortless, breathtaking—and safe—skiing becomes.

This principle of reckless relaxation (anticipation) works similarly in our daily lives as well. The more courageous our faith in God, the more we relax and stop worrying about life's situations. In this posture of anticipation we can enjoy our families and friendships and our service to God. In the spiritual walk as we continue to cultivate the basic mindset of faith and trust in God's love and goodness, life becomes easy in the same way skiing can be easy and fun when we relax and "lean in."

How do we learn to relax and lean in to life, especially when it presents us with difficult challenges? We simply drop to our knees in prayer and commit everything in our lives once again to Christ. Then, when we stand up in courageous faith in God's power to help us, the run on the "ski slope" of our lives is smoother. These challenging "runs" in life become smoother, easier, and more tranquil, and require less energy and less effort. The rest of God fills our hearts and minds with

His peace as we continually yield our lives to Him and trust Him in every life challenge.

> Be strong and courageous. Do not be afraid or terrified because of them, for the LORD your God goes with you; he will never leave you nor forsake you.
>
> —DEUTERONOMY 31:6

Courageous faith says we are filled with God's presence and that is sufficient for us. Out of that faith comes the ability to love, because the Scriptures teach that faith works through love and love works through faith (Gal. 5:6). When we live a life of courageous faith, we are as powerful as a flowing river filled with God's love. We become a wellspring of life to others as they encounter the joy of the Lord inside us and His love flowing out of us.

GIVING COURAGEOUSLY

Giving courageously is one practical way we can express our courageous faith in God. Did you know that when we are generous, we are actually waging spiritual warfare? What we are doing is fighting with "the god of mammon" and showing our allegiance to the God of all creation. When we give away money and possessions to other people in need, we are confirming that God is our source and we are only giving out of His abundance to us.

And giving courageously isn't just about money and possessions. When we appreciate and esteem others as Christ teaches us to do, we will find ways to give His love to them out of our affections. Living a life of courageous faith is reflected in our interaction with others as a *giving* faith. (See James 2:14–17.)

Jesus taught us about giving generously and offering hospitality when He miraculously fed five thousand men from five loaves of bread and two fish. (See Luke 9:10–17.) In this passage we find Jesus with a crowd gathered around Him, as was true so many times during His ministry on earth. As the day wore on, the people grew hungry. There were no food sources in the vicinity, especially to accommodate such a huge crowd. The disciples didn't know what to do. They thought it best to just send the people away. However, Jesus had a plan to demonstrate His generous spirit: "You give them something to eat," He said (v. 13).

All the disciples could find were a few fish and loaves of bread, which they brought to Jesus, lamenting that it was not enough. To begin to feed so many people, Jesus took the loaves of bread and the fish and blessed them, giving thanks to God. Then He instructed the disciples to begin feeding the people. As they did, the bread and fish multiplied until all were fed, with a quantity left over.

Jesus' message is clear: Do what you can with what you have to give to others, giving thanks to God, and God will provide all you need for that situation. When we look to heaven just as Jesus did for supernatural provision, God will provide our physical as well as spiritual needs for abundant life. We have no cause for worry as children of God; we do not need to become covetous and greedy. The Scriptures condemn selfish greed that holds on to what it has and seeks to gain more for itself, which is the opposite of generosity.

If we worry about how we can keep our money and our possessions for ourselves, they will do us no good and will benefit no one. I know many people who give more than they earn, drawing from reserves to meet the needs of others with less. They are generous givers, reflecting the love of God for us, whose inward beings are thankful for what they have and who want to share with others. A giving heart is one that truly appreciates God and others and expresses that appreciation through generosity.

It takes courageous faith to reflect the love of God through courageous giving. It's important to give from our hearts in the joy of the Lord. We can't give solely out of a sense of duty or out of guilt. We can't give in a godly way if our giving is motivated only by a desire to feel proud of ourselves or build ourselves up in the eyes of others. We can genuinely give only when we do so out of courageous faith, knowing God has anointed it for His purposes.

On a practical note, it is also important to evaluate where to give our money. As good stewards in giving we must make sure our gifts go to those who are also good stewards of the funds they receive. We should give to those organizations and individuals where the money will be most efficiently used for the Lord's work, to the greatest benefit, both now and throughout the ensuing years. As we decide where to give our money, we must try to ascertain that Jesus Christ is the center of any ministry to which we consider donating funds. Money should be given with a great deal of discernment through prayer and focusing on the person of Jesus Christ.

Our uneasiness about giving money goes away when we walk in courageous faith, believing that God will be our provider and living in gratitude for all He has given us. Our uneasiness about how those gifts will be used goes away when we pray and listen to the Holy Spirit's direction about where and when to give. When we can give without anxiety in this area of giving, we exhibit our courageous faith in God and demonstrate His love working recklessly in our lives. Others will see the difference that God's love in our lives is making in our generosity and joy in giving. Our trust in God's sovereignty and in His faithfulness helps us to follow His direction in all of our giving.

LOVING COURAGEOUSLY

The Scriptures teach us to "love [our] neighbor as [ourselves]" (Matt. 22:39). This kind of love is a profound reflection of our courageous faith that is based in our love for God. However, it's not so difficult when we learn to appreciate others as being as special to God as we are. Philosophers have divided love into categories. C. S. Lewis wrote about four categories of love in his book *The Four Loves*.[1] First, he defines *love* as *philos*, which is the love shared among friends. Then there is *eros*, which defines love between man and woman. *Agape* is the love God has for us and the love we have for Him. It is the types of love we experience with our friends and family that help us understand the more profound love of God.

The fourth category of love Lewis describes using the word *storge*, which simply means a shared affection. According to Lewis, it's like glue holding the other three loves together. This affection is the humblest love—a love without airs. It binds us together. When its essence enters into the other loves, it is the very medium by which they are reflected from day to day.

Storge relates to our attitude of thanksgiving in which we live our lives. As Lewis discusses *storge*, he also seems to describe it as "appreciation."[2] "In my experience," writes Lewis, "it is affection that creates a [wide] taste [in humanity], teaching us first to notice, then to endure, then to smile at, then to enjoy, and finally to appreciate, the people who 'happen to be there.'"[3] We can't have a constant attitude of thanksgiving without experiencing this simple affection that ultimately leads to appreciation. We appreciate the Lord, not just for everything He does for us but also for who He is, and so we live in thanksgiving in our relationship with Him. And that thanksgiving leads to a profound, intrinsic love relationship with God, which is our internal response to our surrender to Him. Affection will help us fulfill the biblical instruction "In lowliness of mind let each esteem others better than himself" (Phil. 2:3, NKJV).

Affection, or *storge*, shouldn't be confused with the other loves. It's through showing simple affection that we genuinely appreciate, respect, care for, and encourage others. This kind of affection transforms our relationships from an attitude of self-serving to self-giving. No longer are we worried about what we can get for ourselves because affection helps us focus on ways to love others; cultivating *storge* makes life more meaningful, as it creates meaningful relationships. We discover that our relationships are one of life's most beautiful blessings.

These three forms of love—*philos, eros,* and *storge*—create the framework through which *agape*—God's love—can be expressed. Those loves weave together to create a symphony of life leading us to enjoy eternal bliss with God. When we surrender our lives to God, we enter into an intimate, heart relationship with Him. This is not a mental relationship in which we may know and respect Christ. It goes much deeper than that. We are actually in love with Christ! And we begin to grow in grace to maturity in which we express courageous faith in our love for others.

When we are genuinely concerned over the worries and concerns of others, two things happen. First, we are able to help others shoulder their burdens, which in turn helps decrease their fears. Second, we take the focus off ourselves and put it on others in a Christlike fashion, becoming living examples of *storge*—genuine affection and appreciation for others. Our relationships with others can then become filled with *agape* love and help keep us focused on loving God above all and seeking His will. Without godly relationships in which we love courageously, we might revert back to a life of selfishness, which culminates in giving place to a mindset of worry once again.

In all of our relationships, we must show respect for one another, encourage one another, and care for one another. We do this at St. Luke's Cataract and Laser Institute by encouraging our patients and their family members daily. God's Word tells us that love (which would include *storge*) gives us His peace because "Perfect love drives out fear" (1 John 4:18).

Our *agape* love for God, as well as our love for friends and family, is realistic, sacrificial, purposeful, willing, and absolute. As God guides us into a life of courageous love, we guide each other to reflect the love of God in our lives. Our response to our faith in God's love is to love others, respecting them, offering consistent appreciation for who they are and what they do, and helping them to grow in love. This is what courageous faith looks like in a life filled with love.

SERVING COURAGEOUSLY

The Scriptures teach that faith works through love (Gal. 5:6), as I mentioned. It is faith for service to God that is birthed out of our profound love for God. Jesus is the role model for service. He is the perfect servant and the perfect caregiver. At home I have a statue of Him washing the feet of His disciples. It helps me remember His service and shows me how I can follow in His steps. One of the greatest roles in the life of a believer is that of a caregiver and a servant. This expression of love embodies *storge*, the affection that "glues" every facet of love together.

Some physicians I've talked with can't wait to retire from their service in the medical field. I do not echo their sentiments; I never want to quit! I want to be a faithful caregiver for the rest of my life. I see many doctors and nurses who feel as I do, as well as many other people, regardless of their current occupation, who just want to be a servant to others for as long as they are able.

Being a caregiver is about courageous giving, not concerned about receiving for ourselves. We usually receive a deep satisfaction and joy in the process, but that isn't our goal. Giving to others keeps us from selfishness and the worries and fears that result from our self-serving approach to life. Serving others makes us stronger people and strengthens our relationships with others.

Conversely if we focus on our own lives, wanting to be served and lifted up and pampered, we end up focused on what others can do to take care of us and meet our needs. I had an aunt who stayed in bed until 10:00 a.m. every day. She always wanted to be pampered. Yet she was never satisfied with what others did for her. She had the nicest husband in the world; he gave her everything she desired. But I don't think she ever appreciated him. She just ended up dissipating and dying without ever finding the true satisfaction and the beautiful feeling of enjoying a life of service to others.

On the other hand, there's the story of a couple who preferred one another above themselves. They tell this story about how their love for each other resolved. It involved their morning preferences for coffee. The husband liked regular coffee. The wife liked flavored coffee. In their marriage, when the husband awoke first, he made flavored coffee. When the wife awoke first, she made regular coffee. This simple gesture of love and caregiving had a great effect on their love relationship.

There is no greater reward you can receive from your work than the joy that comes from loving service and caregiving. When I see patients, I thank them for letting me be their caregiver. I don't want to be just their physician; I want to be a servant to them. Each of us should strive to be thankful servants to others. Several of us at St. Luke's Cataract and Laser Institute have committed ourselves to recite the thirteenth chapter of 1 Corinthians each day, which is often called the "love chapter." We want to focus on what is so easy to miss in our daily lives—loving the Lord and loving others. The following is a paraphrase of this chapter, substituting words related to love with the term *caregiving*—showing the role of practical love as it meets the road of reality:

> If I speak in the tongues of men and of angels, but have not a caregiver's heart, I am only a resounding gong or a clanging cymbal. Therefore, if I talk about things that are important in medicine, theology and science, but really don't care for people, I'm pretty hollow.
>
> If I have the gift of prophecy and can fathom all mysteries

and all knowledge, and if I have a faith that can move mountains, but have not a caregiver's heart, I am nothing. In other
words, I can be smart and biblical, having been saved by
grace through faith, but if I don't have a caregiver's heart, I'm
nothing.

If I give all I possess to the poor and surrender my body
to the flames, but am not a caregiver, I gain nothing. I can be
generous to others and give sacrificially, but unless my heart
is full of godly love, and I am caring for others, I've missed
my ministry in Christ—for me to focus on Him and, as a
result, be a caregiver.

Caregiving is patient (How I wish I were more patient!),
caregiving is kind. Caregiving does not envy another person's
caregiving or anything else. Envy and covetousness destroy
our relationship with God. He is most satisfied with us when
we are most satisfied with Him. Caregiving does not boast of
caregiving or anything else. Whatever comes, comes...and is
taken as a matter of fact. Caregivers care because they love
Jesus. Caregiving is not proud. Caregiving is humble. The true
caregiver doesn't give care for recognition but cares because
his heart has been changed toward Christ, and he delights in
the ministry of caregiving.

Caregiving is not rude. It does not interrupt. Caregiving
is not self-seeking. It is not done for the benefits the caregiver receives. A caregiver is not easily angered. A caregiver
keeps no record of wrongs. The caregiver keeps focused on
God's grace, His love, His person—and as a result becomes
a caregiver.

A caregiver does not delight in evil but rejoices with the truth,
which is God's love, His life, His light, and His Son.

Caregiving always protects, always trusts. A caregiver
always looks at the best in others and can be depended upon.
A caregiver always hopes for the best and always perseveres in
the caregiving. For example, the Good Samaritan (see Luke
10:25–37) gave freely of his time and money. He was greater
than the priest and the Levite who were interested in their
positions and did not care.

Caregiving never fails. But where there are prophecies and

wisdoms, they will cease; where there are tongues and great orations and talks, they will be stilled; where there is great medical and theological knowledge, it will pass away quickly.

For we know in part, we know a little bit about what is involved in caring for patients and others, and we guess what may come in the future, but when perfection comes, when Christ comes, the imperfect disappears.

When I was a child, throughout my pilgrimage on earth learning to be a better caregiver, I talked like a child, I thought like a child, I reasoned like a child. When I became a man, when I became truly mature, I put childish ways behind me (though those closest to me may not see it sometimes).

Now we see but a poor reflection as in a mirror of the things that are going to come; then we shall see the Lord face to face. Now I know in part about God and theology from the Bible; then I shall know fully, and that is full intimacy, even as I am fully known. As a Christian, I seek God's intimacy more than anything. I need God's intimacy to be a caregiver.

And now these three remain: faith, hope, and caregiving. But the greatest of these is caregiving. It changes us first on the inside and then on the outside. Faith works through love, and hope results from it. Caregiving is the love we show to others in our families, in our social relationships, and in our profession of medicine.

May each of us follow the courageous way of service through this practical expression of loving others. Caregiving is the ultimate expression of love, appreciation, and encouragement. It's the greatest result of *storge* blending with the other categories of love of our lives, shifting our focus from ourselves to others, making us caregivers who have discarded our selfishness for courageous service. When we appreciate others enough to serve them in genuine love and care, we don't have time to worry about ourselves. When we focus on the needs of others, our own selfish needs and desires fade away. When this happens, our hearts can be truly satisfied in our relationship with God, who promises to meet all our needs (Phil. 4:19). And we are filled with the joy of serving God's people as He directs us.

We are transformed inside and out as we learn to trust in God's present and future grace, thus preparing us for a life of bliss throughout eternity with Him. This fundamental transformation of our mindset for life enables us to appreciate God for who He truly is—our constant provider, our agent of change, our Lord and Redeemer, and our heavenly friend. Amen.

DISCUSSION ⚘ QUESTIONS

1. List some ways you can live a life of courageous faith this week.

....

....

....

....

....

2. What keeps you from courageously giving of yourself?

....

....

....

3. Apply *storge* to your relationships with others. How does it change them?

....

....

....

4. Do you know caregivers? Ask them why they serve others.

....

....

....

....

CHAPTER 11

GROWING IN OUR
RELATIONSHIP WITH GOD

WHEN EACH OF us crosses the line, abandoning our self-preservation and committing our lives to the person of Jesus Christ, we are plunged into a process of spiritual transformation: from selfishness to love, from worry and fear to faith, from focusing on ourselves to serving others. We don't always make clear, steady progress on this journey into a deeper relationship with God. Sometimes it's two steps forward and three back. Always we hope that the three steps back are small and that there are more steps forward overall. Yet we must continue our resolve to go through all the challenges life brings as we grow in our intimacy with Christ.

We should never waver in our commitment to His process of transformation. Few things are accomplished immediately. No one can decide one day he will run a marathon the next. He must train diligently for months. It's the same with our spiritual transformation. We cannot be transformed in a day. But we live a life of courageous faith by committing to the process every day.

Life is much like the eighth round of a ten-round fight. We have to keep getting up and getting back in the ring though we have suffered blow after blow in that ring. We might have taken hits in the past; we might have even been knocked down by events. But we need to get up every morning determined to keep going. And we need to let that persistence extend throughout the day, every day, keeping our focus on God despite all the setbacks and disappointments we face from the world.

All of us have times in our lives when we feel up and times when we feel down. Yet we must not let our inner peace be destroyed by outside circumstances and events. In those down times we still need to be filled with thanksgiving as we rest in the wonderful redemption of our Lord. Time spent in His presence, basking in His love and receiving reassurance from His Word as children of God, will strengthen our faith and resolve to pursue relationship with Him at all costs.

When we accept God's call to be His children, we commit ourselves to building an intimate, personal relationship with the person of Jesus Christ. Growing in relationship with God involves receiving new revelation of who He is and discovering His purpose for life. Our praise and thanksgiving expressed to Him keep us strong in the up-and-down cycles as we are being continually transformed by the grace of God into His character, His *agape* love. As believers we're all going through this process of transformation—of focusing on God and not on ourselves. The struggle against selfishness and worry is a continual one. And we can encourage one another as we face situations in life that become catalysts for our growing in our relationship with God.

Throughout history God has been revealing Himself in greater depth for all who will focus on Him. Old Testament saints had revelation of God through their interaction with Him. Enoch, Noah, Abraham, Moses, and others each experienced God in different ways. Their lives teach us who God is and how He desires to interact with His creation— mankind. Then, when Christ came, He taught that His mission was to reveal the heart of the Father to us (see John 14:1–10) and to give His life as a ransom for our sin. Christ is the most perfect revelation of God's *agape* love in the earth.

It is interesting to read in Hebrews 1:1–2 that God made the universe through Christ. In a real sense the phenomenal discoveries that science is making regarding the marvels of the universe are revealing the power and love of God to our generation in ways that have never been known before. Dr. Richard A. Swenson, the author of *More Than Meets the Eye*, astutely observes that "people who lived at the time of Christ enjoyed a special privilege: they looked God in the eye" in the person of Jesus. "While we do not have that physical proximity to Jesus, we have one advantage earlier people lacked"—the revelation of God's power and greatness and love through new discoveries made by science. We can continually grow in our awe and adoration of God as we consider these discoveries of the wonder of the universe that He made. Swenson admits that "science hardly compares to the physical presence of Jesus or the revealed truth of Scripture." Yet we would be wise not to underestimate its power to create deep appreciation in our hearts for our Creator. Science "provides us an advantage in spiritual perspective previous generations could hardly imagine. People of faith often tend to fear science or even dread it. My feeling, however, is quite different."[1]

The knowledge of our Creator that science is giving us is thrilling. "True science is a friend of Truth.... Truthful science, however, always tells us much about the power, precision, design, and sovereignty of God—details we learn nowhere else."[2] Swenson concludes: "God has allowed us the privilege of living in a time when great mysteries of the universe and of mankind are being uncovered. No previous era knew about quantum mechanics, relativity, subatomic particles, supernovas, ageless photons, or DNA. They all reveal the stunning genius of a God who spoke a time-space-matter-light universe into existence, balanced it with impossible requirements of precision, and then gifted it with life.... Science is a close friend of the theology of God's sovereignty. None of these findings were understood in detail until science uncovered them. When science digs, faith rightly grows."[3]

In every way that our relationship with God grows—through studying His Word, through praying, through worshipping, through fellowshipping with other believers, and in learning to appreciate God's greatness in all of creation—we are being transformed into the image of Christ as children of God living in His kingdom.

We should never say we've attained complete transformation of our character while we live on earth. Our relationship with God is not perfected until we join Him in heaven. Our salvation doesn't make us perfect, but it does change our focus and fill our hearts with love for God and for others. The cares and deceits of this world can easily creep in on all of us almost unwittingly. We're still bombarded by the clamor of the world and its lies and agendas. None of us is perfect. As the license plate says, "I'm just getting better through Christ." At best we are believers in a state of repentance learning to take our focus off the world and our own agendas and place it on God's eternal love and His purposes for our lives. Our Christian life is a constant process of focusing and refocusing on eternal values. Praise God, whose grace brings us back to Him from every "detour" in His infinite love and kindness!

We also have a secret weapon that keeps our faith strong: the knowledge that we already have ultimate victory because we read the last page of the Book and we win. We believe in God and His present and future grace, and that is Christ's triumph over sin and death that has given us this ultimate victory (John 16:33). The world can throw all it wants at us; we have the ultimate partner in our corner. We have an intimate, personal relationship with the King of kings and the Lord of lords. We have victory over the world through Jesus Christ!

EMBRACING AN ETERNAL PERSPECTIVE

So with the great victory that is ours in Christ Jesus, why do we still forget at times to be thankful? Why can't we conquer worry? Why does fear so easily overtake us? I believe the answer lies in the fact that we are easily diverted from our focus on God because we continue to look for satisfaction in other areas. That worldly focus lets our minds get cluttered with worldly attitudes, goals, and perspectives rather than the eternal perspective and values of God. When this happens, our appreciation for God falters because we have lost sight of His great faithfulness and His sovereign lordship over our lives. As our appreciation diminishes, our worship and adoration lag, which keeps our heart from where it longs to be—resting in His presence. That is when we need to stir our courageous faith by returning to His presence, waiting on Him to reassure us with His great love.

There's no question that our greatest fulfillment and peace are to be found in the unseen and the eternal through our relationship with God. Yet it's difficult to sustain deep faith and trust at times, so we sacrifice the unseen and the eternal for the very temporary and relatively worthless activities of the present. Maintaining deep faith violates our normal, human way of thinking—of wanting to be independent and self-sufficient, desiring to take care of ourselves. Only as we determine to wait on God will we conquer our natural tendencies to independence.

Remember, God didn't just create the world and set it in motion, then walk away. He was intimately involved in the creation of each of us. That means that He has unsurpassed knowledge of us and is intimately involved in our transformation. In his letter to the Philippians, Paul teaches that "he who began a good work in you will carry it on to completion until the day of Christ Jesus" (Phil. 1:6). God "began a good work" in us. He has started the process, and He will see it through to completion.

In Hebrews 12:1 the author compares this process of transformation with running a race: "Let us run with perseverance the race marked out for us." In the same way a runner prepares for the various conditions possible in a race, God wants us to be prepared for the harsh conditions the world throws at us. He wants us to be ready for the times when we face the hardships, life challenges that threaten us with worry and fear, or desires for the temporal pleasures of the world. With our minds, hearts, and bodies we must continually commit to Him and His training regimen. That transformative training involves our commitment to being *faithful, fervent,* and *focused*. I call these training elements the three Fs.

FAITHFUL

The Book of Revelation declares that one of Christ's names is "Faithful and True" (Rev. 19:11). For believers, being faithful means being aligned to Christ, having faith not in ourselves but in God. Faith is the essence of all our strength in God. Our faith is based in what we know. We know we have a Creator, and by the Word of God we know we have a Redeemer. We are satisfied with all that God is for us in Jesus. In faith we strive to know Him in spirit and evidence Him in our actions. We seek to take on the mind of Christ, rather than hold on to our rebellious, worldly minds.

> I want to know Christ—yes, to know the power of his resurrection.
>
> —PHILIPPIANS 3:10

In this passage in Philippians, Paul talks about "knowing" on an intimate level. For example, in a marriage the partners "know" each other through physical, emotional, and intellectual intimacy.

In that same sort of union with Jesus Christ, everything is found in Him and our total life is committed to Him. We are with Him in our waking and our sleeping. Our lives are lived in prayer and petition; we look to Him and not to ourselves. In fact our very first petition should be that we become intimate with Him so that by living in His presence we will constantly seek His guidance, His wisdom, His knowledge, and His strength. We know that He is real and relevant. We know His power and direction in our lives. We know He sustains us. We know Him as "Faithful and True."

Knowing Him comes through living in God's Word—the Bible. We have to be with God in the Word through the power of the Holy Spirit to grow spiritually and to carry out His work. When the Word of God dwells in us richly, the Spirit takes that Word and makes it part of us, transforming our minds as it shapes our desires, our focus, and our leanings.

I encourage you to memorize Scripture and then use that Scripture in your life and prayers. When we fill ourselves with the Word of God, meditating on Scripture every day and seeking the Lord through His Word, He will give us a mindset of peace. With the Word in us our prayers become more focused. We can pray the Word back to the Lord, inserting our names as the Spirit leads. The power of the living Word of God in us enables us to plant our feet firmly on earth and stand on His claims that are written about us as His children.

> You will keep in perfect peace those whose minds are steadfast, because they trust in you.
>
> —ISAIAH 26:3

In this verse Isaiah was implying that he had peace when he heard God's Word and trusted in it, rather than trusting in his own intelligence. This was no small feat. Isaiah may have been one of the most intelligent men of the Old Testament. It may have taken a great deal of effort, will, and commitment for him to trust God first, rather than his own intellect. Isaiah's faithfulness was essential to his transformation.

If we are to have perfect peace, our minds must be fixed on God and His kingdom and not on the world. Devoting time every day to reading the Bible helps us do this. We are the soil into which God's Holy Spirit will sow His Word. One of the best ways to get the Word of God into every part of our lives is by memorizing verses. In fact it is wisdom to know and memorize Scripture.

Often I have merely read Scripture without perceiving or receiving its meaning and truth. Conversely I can meditate for days and days, for years and years, on one word in the Bible. We must truly meditate on the Word and have that Word dictate the thoughts of our hearts so that every word of God sown into us gives a hundredfold return.

God desires that we follow His direction in Scripture as a way of life. In doing so, His kingdom advances through us. This means that every day, we must proclaim the Word of God, the truth of God. We must pray it, say it, believe it, and live it. That is the only way to be faithful. However, we are always conscious that our trust is in His faithfulness, not ours! He is faithful, and relying on Him stirs us up to be faithful.

FERVENT

Faith both fuels and is strengthened by our passion—fervent desire and inner longing—for intimacy with God. We must have the desire to be focused on and aligned with Christ in a way that truly makes us want to be healed from all the evils of the world. That desire includes healing from worry and living in a thanksgiving frenzy. It's a passionate cry of focusing on the Lord.

> As the deer pants for streams of water, so my soul pants for
> you, my God. My soul thirsts for God, for the living God.
> —PSALM 42:1–2

We are called to surrender to God not out of duty but out of love, fervent love that springs from the knowledge of His great love for us through Jesus Christ. As we love Him, embracing Him with our whole being and seeking His presence in our lives through intimate relationship, God's grace makes us more like Jesus Christ. As we are conformed more and more into the image of His Son, our desires yield to His desires.

We must fervently desire to be transformed; we must fervently desire to be more Christlike. We can't just know in our heads who Christ is and how to be like Him. We must have a fervent desire in our hearts to be *like* Him. It is fervency that transforms us. As we love God and are in love with Him, we're overwhelmed with thanksgiving and joy.

> Sing and make music from your heart to the Lord, always
> giving thanks to God the Father for everything, in the name
> of our Lord Jesus Christ.
> —EPHESIANS 5:19–20

If all we desire are the things of this world, we'll fail. We will fall victim to selfishness, to our independent spirits. It is our passion for the living God that keeps us close to Him. When love is present in a marriage, it's much easier to keep the relationship on track. When we find love in our relationship with God, growing close to Him is easier. We're lifted off this earth and freed from the cares of this world until we are engulfed in His presence as we stand fast in His promises.

FOCUSED

To be transformed, to become Christlike, we must be focused on Him, refusing to be distracted, never looking back or to the left or the right. Our focus must be on Christ alone if we are to be transformed. I have a cousin who is very bright. He was always quite successful in school, even medical school. He once told me that the secret to medical school for him was not his intelligence. It was his diligence. He said, "You know, the difference between those who made it and those who didn't was diligence. Those who failed were quitters; they weren't dedicated enough to keep on going."

Persistence is crucial to success. Satan knows this. That is why he works hard to get us off track, off the path God has for us. If he can replace humility with pride, he has us. He would love for us to start feeling proud of how well we're doing in our relationships with God, to think we have enough passion and faith to get through. He would love for us to think it's OK to stay where we are, that we don't need to grow any further. In fact he would love it if, because we're doing so well, we start to think we don't need God quite as much. When that happens, we start slipping back into our independent, selfish natures, comparing ourselves with others, worrying about whether we have everything we need. We take our eyes off God and start noticing the things of the world.

The process of transformation takes persistence. It calls for us to be stubborn in our faith, stubborn in our desire, and stubborn in our determination that nothing can shake us from our focus on God, who loves us. He is faithful in His provision for us, and nothing can separate us from His love. There is no other way for us to respond to Him than with that same determination, based in love, joy, and thanksgiving. It is a godly perspective of life at all times that will give us that kind of determination. God's perspective helps us appreciate the life of Him who dwells in us. When compared with the temporal pleasures and possessions of this life, our eternal perspective is ultimately of much more worth. It keeps us from becoming discouraged even in difficult times.

None of us should ever give up. We should never say we've attained perfect transformation. It is through God's grace that we grow closer to Him through His Son, Jesus Christ. The final form of the kingdom of God lies ahead of us. Until then we wait for Him, we work for Him, we live with Jesus in our hearts, and we will see what God does through us as we go forward in faith.

When we turn our total being away from worry, when we trust in God's grace and get rid of all the worldly distractions, when we live in a thanksgiving frenzy, we are wrapped up in a cloud of exuberance that transcends this world. This process of transformation keeps us focused so that when we are ultimately translated into God's presence in heaven, we'll find our exuberance multiplied immeasurably.

DISCUSSION QUESTIONS

1. Do you worry more or worry less than you did when you were younger? Do you worry about the same things?

....

....

....

....

2. List some ways you can practice being faithful to Christ this week.

....

....

....

....

3. How can you grow personally in your relationship with God? How do you feel passion for God's presence?

....

....

....

....

4. What obstacles keep you from being focused on the Lord? Describe some ways you can overcome them this week.

....

....

....

PUTTING PROMISES
INTO ACTION

A RE YOU WORRIED about a specific relationship or circumstance? This appendix lists some key Bible verses you can use to battle worry and fear. These verses are God's promises to believers that He is with us and will be our support and strength. Read them. Believe them. Let His Word become the foundation in your struggles!

Are you worried, anxious, afraid, or troubled? God will give you peace.

In my distress I called to the LORD; I cried to my God for help. From his temple he heard my voice; my cry came before him, into his ears....He brought me out into a spacious place; he rescued me because he delighted in me.

—PSALM 18:6, 19

God is our refuge and strength, an ever-present help in trouble. Therefore we will not fear, though the earth give way and the mountains fall into the heart of the sea.

—PSALM 46:1–2

When I am afraid, I put my trust in you. In God, whose word I praise—in God I trust and am not afraid. What can mere mortals do to me?

—Psalm 56:3–4

You will keep in perfect peace those whose minds are steadfast, because they trust in you.

—Isaiah 26:3

Do not let your hearts be troubled. You believe in God; believe also in me.... Peace I leave with you; my peace I give you. I do not give to you as the world gives. Do not let your hearts be troubled and do not be afraid.

—John 14:1, 27

I have told you these things, so that in me you may have peace. In this world you will have trouble. But take heart! I have overcome the world.

—John 16:33

Do not be anxious about anything, but in every situation, by prayer and petition, with thanksgiving, present your requests to God. And the peace of God, which transcends all understanding, will guard your hearts and your minds in Christ Jesus.

—Philippians 4:6–7

Are you worried about the future? God will guide you.

He guides the humble in what is right and teaches them his way.

—Psalm 25:9

I will instruct you and teach you in the way you should go; I will counsel you with my loving eye on you.

—Psalm 32:8

The LORD makes firm the steps of the one who delights in him; though he may stumble, he will not fall, for the LORD upholds him with his hand.

—PSALM 37:23–24

Trust in the LORD with all your heart and lean not on your own understanding; in all your ways submit to him, and he will make your paths straight.

—PROVERBS 3:5–6

Commit to the LORD whatever you do, and he will establish your plans.

—PROVERBS 16:3

So do not fear, for I am with you; do not be dismayed, for I am your God. I will strengthen you and help you; I will uphold you with my righteous right hand.

—ISAIAH 41:10

"For I know the plans I have for you," declares the LORD, "plans to prosper you and not to harm you, plans to give you hope and a future."

—JEREMIAH 29:11

If any of you lacks wisdom, you should ask God, who gives generously to all without finding fault, and it will be given to you.

—JAMES 1:5

Are you afraid of feeling alone? God will never leave you.

Be strong and courageous. Do not be afraid or terrified because of them, for the LORD your God goes with you; he will never leave you nor forsake you.

—DEUTERONOMY 31:6

Then you will call, and the LORD will answer; you will cry for help, and he will say: Here am I.

—ISAIAH 58:9

The LORD your God is with you, the Mighty Warrior who saves. He will take great delight in you; in his love he will no longer rebuke you, but will rejoice over you with singing.

—ZEPHANIAH 3:17

I will not leave you as orphans; I will come to you.

—JOHN 14:18

Are you worried no one loves you? God loves you.

For God so loved the world that he gave his one and only Son, that whoever believes in him shall not perish but have eternal life.

—JOHN 3:16

For I am convinced that neither death nor life, neither angels nor demons, neither the present nor the future, nor any powers, neither height nor depth, nor anything else in all creation, will be able to separate us from the love of God that is in Christ Jesus our Lord.

—ROMANS 8:38–39

This is how we know what love is: Jesus Christ laid down his life for us. And we ought to lay down our lives for our brothers and sisters.

—1 JOHN 3:16

This is love: not that we loved God, but that he loved us and sent his Son as an atoning sacrifice for our sins.

—1 JOHN 4:10

Are you worried that God could never forgive your sins? God's salvation overcomes all sins and guilt.

As far as the east is from the west, so far has he removed our transgressions from us.

—PSALM 103:12

If we confess our sins, he is faithful and just and will forgive us our sins and purify us from all unrighteousness.

—1 JOHN 1:9

Do you feel depressed? God will comfort you.

The LORD is close to the brokenhearted and saves those who are crushed in spirit.

—PSALM 34:18

Why, my soul, are you downcast? Why so disturbed within me? Put your hope in God, for I will yet praise him, my Savior and my God.

—PSALM 42:11

Are you worried because you face opposition? God is with you.

If God is for us, who can be against us?

—ROMANS 8:31

Are you worried about physical needs? God will provide.

Therefore I tell you, do not worry about your life, what you will eat or drink; or about your body, what you will wear. Is not life more than food, and the body more than clothes? Look at the birds of the air; they do not sow or reap or store away in barns, and yet your heavenly Father feeds them. Are you not much more valuable than they? Can any one of you by worrying add a single hour to your life?

And why do you worry about clothes? See how the flowers of the field grow. They do not labor or spin. Yet I tell you that not even Solomon in all his splendor was dressed like one of these. If that is how God clothes the grass of the field, which is here today and tomorrow is thrown into the fire, will he not much more clothe you—you of little faith? So do not worry, saying, "What shall we eat?" or "What shall we drink?" or "What shall we wear?" For the pagans run after all these things, and your heavenly Father knows that you need them.

But seek first his kingdom and his righteousness, and all these things will be given to you as well. Therefore do not worry about tomorrow, for tomorrow will worry about itself. Each day has enough trouble of its own.

—MATTHEW 6:25–34

If you, then, though you are evil, know how to give good gifts to your children, how much more will your Father in heaven give good gifts to those who ask him!

—MATTHEW 7:11

Are not five sparrows sold for two pennies? Yet not one of them is forgotten by God. Indeed, the very hairs of your head are all numbered. Don't be afraid; you are worth more than many sparrows.

—LUKE 12:6–7

He who did not spare his own Son, but gave him up for us all—how will he not also, along with him, graciously give us all things?

—ROMANS 8:32

And God is able to bless you abundantly, so that in all things at all times, having all that you need, you will abound in every good work.

—2 CORINTHIANS 9:8

And my God will meet all your needs according to the riches of his glory in Christ Jesus.

—PHILIPPIANS 4:19

Do you worry about your safety? God will protect you.

In peace I will lie down and sleep, for you alone, LORD, make me dwell in safety.

—PSALM 4:8

The LORD will keep you from all harm—he will watch over your life; the LORD will watch over your coming and going both now and forevermore.

—PSALM 121:7–8

Do you worry so much that you can't sleep? God will ease your fears.

I lie down and sleep; I wake again, because the LORD sustains me.

—PSALM 3:5

In peace I will lie down and sleep, for you alone, LORD, make me dwell in safety.

—PSALM 4:8

When you lie down, you will not be afraid; when you lie down, your sleep will be sweet.

—PROVERBS 3:24

Are you worried about your appearance? God looks at your heart.

But the LORD said to Samuel, "Do not consider his appearance or his height, for I have rejected him. The LORD does not look at the things people look at. People look at the outward appearance, but the LORD looks at the heart."

—1 SAMUEL 16:7

He has made everything beautiful in its time. He has also set eternity in the human heart; yet no one can fathom what God has done from beginning to end.

—ECCLESIASTES 3:11

Are you worried about your health? God will give you strength.

The righteous person may have many troubles, but the LORD delivers him from them all.

—PSALM 34:19

The LORD will guide you always; he will satisfy your needs in a sun-scorched land and will strengthen your frame.

—ISAIAH 58:11

"But I will restore you to health and heal your wounds," declares the LORD, "because you are called an outcast, Zion for whom no one cares."

—JEREMIAH 30:17

Is anyone among you sick? Let them call the elders of the church to pray over them and anoint them with oil in the name of the Lord. And the prayer offered in faith will make the sick person well; the Lord will raise them up.

—JAMES 5:14–15

Are you worried about getting old? God will stay with you.

The righteous will flourish like a palm tree, they will grow like a cedar of Lebanon; planted in the house of the LORD, they will flourish in the courts of our God. They will still bear fruit in old age, they will stay fresh and green.

—PSALM 92:12–14

Even to your old age and gray hairs I am he, I am he who will sustain you.

—ISAIAH 46:4

Are you worried about dying? God offers eternal life.

Even though I walk through the darkest valley, I will fear no evil, for you are with me; your rod and your staff, they comfort me.

—PSALM 23:4

For God so loved the world that he gave his one and only Son, that whoever believes in him shall not perish but have eternal life.

—JOHN 3:16

I give them eternal life, and they shall never perish; no one will snatch them out of my hand.

—JOHN 10:28

"Where, O death, is your victory? Where, O death, is your sting?"... Thanks be to God! He gives us the victory through our Lord Jesus Christ.

—1 CORINTHIANS 15:55, 57

Since the children have flesh and blood, he too shared in their humanity so that by his death he might break the power of him who holds the power of death—that is, the devil—and free those who all their lives were held in slavery by their fear of death.

—HEBREWS 2:14–15

ABOUT
THE AUTHOR

J AMES P. GILLS, MD, received his medical degree from Duke University Medical Center in 1959. He served his ophthalmology residency at Wilmer Ophthalmological Institute of Johns Hopkins University from 1962 to 1965. Dr. Gills founded the St. Luke's Cataract and Laser Institute in Tarpon Springs, Florida, and has performed more cataract and lens implant surgeries than any other eye surgeon in the world. Since establishing his Florida practice in 1968, he has been firmly committed to embracing new technology and perfecting the latest cataract surgery techniques. In 1974, he became the first eye surgeon in the United States to dedicate his practice to cataract treatment through the use of intraocular lenses. Dr. Gills has been recognized in Florida and throughout the world for his professional accomplishments and personal commitment to helping others. He has been recognized by the readers of *Cataract & Refractive Surgery Today* as one of the top fifty cataract and refractive opinion leaders.

As a world-renowned ophthalmologist, Dr. Gills has received innumerable medical and educational awards and has been listed in *The Best Doctors in America*. As a clinical professor of ophthalmology at the University of South Florida, he was named one of the best ophthalmologists in America in 1996 by ophthalmic academic leaders nationwide. He has served on the board of directors of the American College of Eye Surgeons, the board of visitors at Duke University Medical Center, and the advisory board of Wilmer Ophthalmological Institute at Johns Hopkins University.

While Dr. Gills has many accomplishments and varied interests, his primary focus is to restore physical vision to patients and to bring spiritual enlightenment through his life. Guided by his strong and enduring faith in Jesus Christ, he seeks to encourage and comfort the patients who come to St. Luke's and to share his faith whenever possible. It was through sharing his insights with patients that he initially began writing on Christian topics. An avid student of the Bible for many years, he has authored numerous books on Christian living, with over nine million copies in print. With the exception of the Bible, Dr. Gills' books are perhaps the most widely requested books in the US prison system. They have been supplied to over two thousand prisons and jails, including every death row facility in the nation. In addition, Dr. Gills has published more than 195 medical articles and has authored or coauthored ten medical reference textbooks. Six of those books were best sellers at the American Academy of Ophthalmology annual meetings.

Did You Enjoy This Book?
We at Love Press would be pleased to hear from you if
God's Rx for Fear and Worry
has had an effect on your life or the lives of your loved ones.
Send your letters to:
Love Press
P.O. Box 1608
Tarpon Springs, FL 34688-1608

NOTES

INTRODUCTION

1. *Merriam-Webster*, s.v. "appreciate," accessed March 6, 2019, https://www.merriam-webster.com/dictionary/appreciate.

CHAPTER 1

1. Charles Horace Mayo, *Aphorisms of Dr. Charles Horace Mayo, 1865–1939, and Dr. William James Mayo, 1861–1939* (Springfield, IL: Charles C. Thomas, 1951).
2. James P. Gills, *God's Prescription for Healing* (Lake Mary, FL: Siloam, 2004), 120. Additional resource: J. T. and Ruth Seamands, *Engineered for Glory* (Wilmore, KY: Francis Asbury Society, 1984).

CHAPTER 2

1. Ellen Vaughn, *Radical Gratitude* (Grand Rapids, MI: Zondervan, 2005), 140.
2. Vaughn, *Radical Gratitude*, 138.

CHAPTER 3

1. Richard Swenson, *More Than Meets the Eye*, DVD presentation (Bristol, TN: Christian Medical and Dental Associations, 2005), www.cmda.org.
2. Swenson, *More Than Meets the Eye*.
3. Swenson, *More Than Meets the Eye*.
4. Isaac Asimov, "In the Game of Energy and Thermodynamics You Can't Even Break Even," *Smithsonian Institute Journal* (June 1970): 10.
5. "Human Brain Can Store 4.7 Billion Books—Ten Times More Than Originally Thought," *Telegraph*, January 21, 2016, https://

www.telegraph.co.uk/news/science/science-news/12114150/
Human-brain-can-store-4.7-billion-books-ten-times-more-
than-originally-thought.html?utm_source=dlvr.it&utm_
medium=twitter.

6. "The Thermodynamics of Brains and Computers," Duke
Department of Physics, accessed March 11, 2019, http://
webhome.phy.duke.edu/~hsg/363/table-images/brain-vs-
computer.html.

7. Carl Zimmer, "How Many Cells Are in Your Body?" *National
Geographic*, October 23, 2013, https://www.nationalgeographic.
com/science/phenomena/2013/10/23/how-many-cells-are-in-
your-body/.

8. Swenson, *More Than Meets the Eye*.

9. Swenson, *More Than Meets the Eye*.

10. Swenson, *More Than Meets the Eye*.

11. *Westminster Shorter Catechism* 1, http://www.
westminsterconfession.org/confessional-standards/the-
westminster-shorter-catechism.php.

CHAPTER 4

1. Gills, *God's Prescription for Healing*.

2. Gills, *God's Prescription for Healing*.

3. Gills, *God's Prescription for Healing*.

4. Gills, *God's Prescription for Healing*.

5. Mark Twain, *Pudd'nhead Wilson* (Mineola, NY: Dover
Publications, 1999), 60.

6. David Jeremiah, *Slaying the Giants in Your Life* (Nashville:
Thomas Nelson, 2001), 4, https://books.google.com/
books?id=RqcVPHpPheQC&pg.

7. Brother Lawrence, *The Practice of the Presence of God and the
Spiritual Maxims* (Mineola, NY: Dover Publications, 2005),
https://books.google.com/books?id=ZBwHwCVtQfsC&.

8. Lawrence, *The Practice of the Presence of God and the Spiritual
Maxims*.

9. Gills, *God's Prescription for Healing*.

10. Gills, *God's Prescription for Healing*.

11. Gills, *God's Prescription for Healing*.

CHAPTER 5

1. *The American Heritage Dictionary of the English Language*, 3rd ed. (Boston: Houghton Mifflin Company, 1992).
2. Martin Luther, *Three Treatises* (Philadelphia: Fortress Press, 1960).
3. Eberhard Bethge, *Dietrich Bonhoeffer* (New York: Harper and Row, 1970).

CHAPTER 6

1. "Barbara W. Tuchman Quotes," BrainyQuote, accessed March 11, 2019, https://www.brainyquote.com/quotes/barbara_w_tuchman_134575.

CHAPTER 7

1. "Mother Teresa Quotes," BrainyQuote, accessed March 12, 2019, https://www.brainyquote.com/quotes/mother_teresa_131834.
2. "Blaise Pascal Quotes," Goodreads, accessed March 12, 2019, https://www.goodreads.com/quotes/801132-there-is-a-god-shaped-vacuum-in-the-heart-of-each.

CHAPTER 8

1. Swenson, *More Than Meets the Eye*, 115. [Robert Wearner, "Newton: Man of the Future," *Signs of the Times*, February 1999, 27; quoting I. Bernard Cohen, "Isaac Newton's Papers and Letters on Natural Philosophy," 928].
2. Swenson, *More Than Meets the Eye*, 114.
3. George Mueller, *Autobiography of George Mueller* (London: J. Nisbet and Co., 1906).

CHAPTER 9

1. Archie P. McDonald, *William Barrett Travis: A Biography* (Austin, TX: Eakins Press, 1976).

CHAPTER 10

1. C. S. Lewis, *The Four Loves* (NY: Harcourt Brace & Company, 1960).
2. Lewis, *The Four Loves*.
3. Lewis, *The Four Loves*.

CHAPTER 11

1. Swenson, *More Than Meets the Eye*, 184.
2. Swenson, *More Than Meets the Eye*, 184–185.
3. Swenson, *More Than Meets the Eye*, 185.